Critical Care Focus

7: Nutritional Issues

EDITOR
DR HELEN F GALLEY
Senior lecturer in Anaesthesia and Intensive Care
University of Aberdeen

EDITORIAL BOARD
PROFESSOR NIGEL R WEBSTER
Professor of Anaesthesia and Intensive Care
University of Aberdeen

DR PAUL G P LAWLER
Clinical Director of Intensive Care
South Cleveland Hospital

DR NEIL SONI
Consultant in Anaesthesia and Intensive Care
Chelsea and Westminster Hospital

DR MERVYN SINGER
Reader in Intensive Care
University College Hospital, London

BMJ
Books

© BMJ Books 2001
BMJ Books is an imprint of the BMJ Publishing Group

First published in 2001
by BMJ Books, BMA House, Tavistock Square,
London WC1H 9JR

www.bmjbooks.com
www.ics.ac.uk

British Library Cataloguing in Publication Data

A catalogue record for this book is available from the British Library

ISBN 0-7279-1652-1

The chapters in this book are based on presentations given at the Intensive Care
Society Focus Meeting on Nutrition, London, November 2000.

Typeset by Newgen Imaging Systems (P) Ltd., Chennai
Printed and bound by Selwood Printing Ltd., West Sussex

Contents

Critical Care Focus series

Also available:

H F Galley (ed) Critical Care Focus 1: *Renal Failure*, 1999.

H F Galley (ed) Critical Care Focus 2: *Respiratory Failure*, 1999.

H F Galley (ed) Critical Care Focus 3: *Neurological Injury*, 2000.

H F Galley (ed) Critical Care Focus 4: *Endocrine Disturbance*, 2000.

H F Galley (ed) Critical Care Focus 5: *Antibiotic Resistance and Infection Control*, 2001.

H F Galley (ed) Critical Care Focus 6: *Cardiology in Critical Illness*, 2001.

Contributors

Simon P Allison
Professor of Clinical Nutrition and Consultant Physician, University Hospital, Queen's Medical Centre, Nottingham, UK, and Chairman of the European Society of Enteral and Parenteral Nutrition

Richard D Griffiths
Reader in Intensive Care Medicine, University of Liverpool and Consultant Physician, Whiston Hospital, St Helen's and Knowsley Hospitals NHS Trust, UK

George K Grimble
Reader in Clinical Nutrition, University of Surrey, UK

Robert F Grimble
Professor of Nutrition, Institute of Human Nutrition, University of Southampton, UK

Paul A O'Toole
Consultant Gastroenterologist, Aintree Hospital, Liverpool, UK

Christopher R Pennington
Clinical Director, Medicine and Cardiovascular Group, Ninewells Hospital, Dundee, UK

Alan Shenkin
Professor of Clinical Chemistry, University of Liverpool and Honorary Consultant in Chemical Pathology, Royal Liverpool and Broadgreen Hospitals NHS Trust, Liverpool, UK and Chairman of the Intercollegiate Group for Nutrition

Duncan L Wyncoll
Consultant in Intensive Care, Guy's and St Thomas' NHS Trust, London, UK

Preface to the Critical Care Focus series

The Critical Care Focus series aims to provide a snapshot of current thoughts and practice, by renowned experts. The complete series should provide a comprehensive guide for all health professionals on key issues in today's field of critical care. The volumes are deliberately concise and easy to read, designed to inform and provoke. Most chapters are produced from transcriptions of lectures at the Intensive Care Society meetings and represent the views of world leaders in their fields.

Helen F Galley

Introduction

Why feed the critically ill patient?

Christopher R Pennington

There are several perhaps obvious reasons why critically ill patients should be fed, and there are also reasons why feeding patients before they reach the stage of critical illness should be considered. Nutritional events which occur early in the progress of illness will determine responses to treatment and may even determine requirement for intensive care in hospital; nutritional events that occur in hospital will determine the extent and length of recovery subsequently. This article will, I hope, convince you that nutritional support does make a difference in the critically ill and why we should indeed feed critically ill patients.

What should we be feeding?

George K Grimble

Malnutrition is a common and often under-recognised problem in hospital patients. Continuing illness and hospitalisation commonly result in negative energy balance and consequently further deterioration in nutritional status. The high prevalence and potentially deleterious effects of such malnutrition have resulted in many trials of the effects of nutritional supplementation in various patient groups. There is much confusing evidence and although some nutritional approaches seem tempting there are few convincing clinical trials and we are forced to the conclusion that we should be performing better clinical trials to get rid of the placebo affect. Study design is clearly paramount. There are interesting new data on immunonutrition and a recent meta-analysis suggests they may indeed affect outcome.

What route?

Paul A O'Toole

This article will discuss the routes which are available for feeding critically ill patients in the intensive care unit. There are few studies addressing this issue and meta-analysis is difficult since there are many differences in the way feeds were given, for example, total parenteral nutrition (TPN) versus enteral nutrition; TPN as a supplement to enteral feeding; the timing of feeding; differences in terms of the patient populations; and pre-existing nutritional state. There are a lot of different options for routes of feeding—this article will discuss those options and try and encourage those feeding critically ill patients to make informed decisions.

Timing of feeding

Simon P Allison

In critically ill patients on the intensive care unit and elsewhere, all the evidence suggests that early feeding, especially in those patients who are malnourished, improves outcome. However, we should not confine our attention just to the time spent on the intensive care unit, since the whole natural history of the patient's condition is important. What we do early on may affect what happens later in the patient's progress, and what we do in anticipation may also improve outcome. The effects of nutritional intervention in the intensive care unit may also not be seen until much later.

Immunonutrition

Robert F Grimble

The systemic inflammatory response which occurs as a result of surgery, trauma or infection may exert high metabolic demands upon patients and lead to a depletion of essential nutrient stores. Cytokines orchestrate the host response to injury and infection and are crucial for normal immune responses. Malnourished patients have a reduced capacity for cytokine production. This article describes the modulatory role that nutrients exert on cytokine biology, and the therapeutic strategies—termed immunonutrition—that are available to counteract these effects.

Glutamine

Richard D Griffiths

Glutamine is synthesised and released from skeletal muscle in the systemic circulation where it acts as an inter-organ nitrogen- and carbon-transporter for intra-cellular glutamate. It is an important energy source both directly, and indirectly by promotion of gluconeogenesis. It is fundamental for protein synthesis where it donates nitrogen for the synthesis of purines, pyrimidines and nucleotides. It is necessary for antioxidants protection via glutathione, and is important for immune function including T helper cell responses and monocyte function. During critical illness, depletion of glutamate may limit these functions and may have an adverse effect on outcome. This article will address the importance of glutamine, and whether exogenous supply of glutamine in the critically ill is beneficial.

Immunonutrition with commercial formulae

Duncan L Wyncoll

Manipulation of the immune and inflammatory responses through nutritional approaches has been termed immunonutrition. Three major groups of so-called immune nutrients have been used, including amino acids such as arginine and glutamine, fatty acids, particularly the omega 3 fatty acids, and purine nucleotides, in the form of yeast RNA. These nutrients have been combined in commercial preparations for enteral feeding, and the evidence of any benefit of feeding these formulae rather than standard formulae to critically ill patients forms the basis of this article.

Micronutrients

Alan Shenkin

The trace element and vitamin requirements (micronutrients) of severely ill or injured patients depend on a complex interaction of the status of the patient at the time of admission, ongoing losses and the potential benefit of supplying large amounts of individual micronutrients. Characteristic clinical deficiency states are now relatively uncommon, but sub-clinical deficiency is of growing concern. The main effects of sub-clinical deficiency include alteration of the balance between reactive oxygen species and antioxidants, leading to oxidative damage of polyunsaturated fatty acids and nucleic acids, and possibly to increased activation of the transcription factor nuclear factor kappa B. This leads to increased production of cytokines and impaired immune function with increased likelihood of infectious complications. Recent studies have indicated the clinical benefit of providing large amounts of certain micronutrients in burned and head injured patients. Further clinical studies are now required to define optimal levels of provision in different disease states, with a particular emphasis on markers of tissue function and clinical outcome.

1: Why feed the critically ill patient?

CHRISTOPHER R PENNINGTON

Introduction

There are several perhaps obvious reasons why critically ill patients should be fed, and there are also reasons why feeding patients before they reach the stage of critical illness should be considered. Patients undertake what could be termed a "journey". During this journey the patients develop symptoms, they go to the clinic and undergo various investigations, their illness is diagnosed, they are admitted to hospital, undergo evaluation, undergo surgery, go to the critical care unit and hopefully recover enough to return to the ward and are discharged and then gradually convalesce. Some of the patients' time is spent in the intensive care unit (ICU) and some of their time is in hospital. A very great deal of time is spent in the community. Patients' journeys are very long and this is important from the nutritional point of view. Nutritional events that occur early in the progress of illness will determine responses to treatment and may even determine requirement for intensive care in hospital. Nutritional events that occur in hospital will determine the extent and length of subsequent recovery.[1,2] This chapter will, hopefully, convince you that nutritional support does make a difference in the critically ill and why we should indeed feed critically ill patients.

Pre-existing nutritional state

It is known that patients deteriorate nutritionally long before they are admitted to hospital. There have been many studies investigating nutritional status in various patient groups on admission to hospital, and some relatively large studies have been undertaken over the last 20 years, which include general medical patients, general surgical patients, patients undergoing orthopaedic surgery, elderly patents and patients in the respiratory medicine unit. Three points need to be made about these data. The first is that the population has become heavier and in essence the goal

1

posts have changed. Secondly, in the more recent studies only some of the less ill patients were investigated—the sicker patients were not investigated. Thirdly, apart from the patients with low body weight, it is clear that patients who have a high body mass index (BMI) and a normal BMI will also have lost weight and weight loss is probably a more important determinant than BMI.

Malnutrition is very common in patients who are admitted to hospital and indeed this not only relates to protein-energy malnutrition, but also involves micronutrient malnutrition and thus antioxidant status, which will determine the extent of tissue injury in the context of critical illness. Furthermore, we know that once patients are admitted to hospital nutritional deterioration continues in two-thirds of them. Nutritional deterioration does occur in those patients who are in hospital for more than a week and we know that the deterioration is particularly common and more severe in those patients who were nutritionally depleted on admission.[3]

There is an assumption that once patients have been treated they get better, and of course they do, but they may not get better immediately from a nutritional perspective. In a recent study in which this author was involved, patients who had undergone abdominal surgery were followed up when they returned into the community.[4] It was found that those patients who had borderline nutritional status postoperatively, continued to deteriorate nutritionally for 8 weeks, had become static by 10 weeks and showed no evidence of recovery in the absence of intervention.

Consequences of malnutrition

In summary therefore, it is clear that the picture in many patients is one of nutritional decline before admission, during admission, and after admission, and this can, of course, have major consequences for the patient.

There are many causes of protein-energy malnutrition including organ failure, immobility, and nutrition. Nutrition has both a direct impact through the prevention of starvation, and an indirect impact through the provision of specific nutrients and antioxidants. This chapter will address the direct impact, which of course relates to starvation. Patients who are critically ill cannot eat; they may starve because food is unavailable, or because they have impaired ingestion due to neurological or other problems. They may also have impaired absorption and, regardless of the reason, patients literally starve. Studies conducted in hospital in the acute setting confirm that patients do indeed starve, since many of the studies reveal that recommended food intakes are commonly not met.[3]

Clearly starvation is an important issue because ultimately it kills patients—we know that in normal subjects who starve, deaths start to occur at around 60–70 days of complete starvation, as shown with hunger strikers. However the situation is different in critically ill patients in several respects. First of all these patients are not normal—many of them are malnourished on admission to hospital and many patients have a metabolic response to injury under the influence of cytokines or disease and therefore decline more rapidly.

Another problem became apparent in a study of conscientious objectors, who were invited to participate in a study of semi-starvation, and it was found that it takes a very long time, many weeks or months, for starving subjects to return to normal. Intervention should therefore be early, and this is particularly true for critically ill patients because it is not possible to prevent, let alone restore to normal, nutritional deterioration in patients who are metabolically stressed.

Reasons to intervene

In a study by Shaw et al.,[5] rates of whole-body protein synthesis and catabolism in normal volunteers and in a group of severely septic patients were isotopically determined. In addition, the effect in the patients of either glucose infusion or total parenteral nutrition (TPN) on protein dynamics was assessed. The basal rate of net protein catabolism was significantly higher in the septic patients than in the volunteers, primarily due to an increase in whole-body catabolism that was partially counteracted by a modest increase in protein synthesis. When the patients were infused with glucose (4 mg/kg/min), net protein catabolism decreased significantly and during TPN the value was significantly lower again. In each instance the conservation of host tissue was due to an increase in protein synthesis: the accelerated rate of whole-body protein catabolism continued irrespective of the nutritional status. The following conclusions were reached from these data: (i) severely ill septic patients have an accelerated rate of net protein catabolism compared with normal volunteers, and this is primarily due to a large increase in whole-body protein catabolism; (ii) TPN is an effective means of conserving host tissue in severely septic patients via the promotion of whole-body protein synthesis; (iii) despite the beneficial effect of TPN in these patients, whole-body protein catabolism continues unabated, and as a result, protein losses still occur at approximately 25% of the rate seen in the absence of TPN; (iv) and there is no obvious advantage in terms of protein-sparing when protein is provided in amounts exceeding 1·5g/kg/day.

There is another important reason why intervention in terms of nutrition should be undertaken early—organ function. For example muscle function is markedly affected by nutritional status. Jeejeebhoy reported, in a study in 1988,[6] that both subjects who are obese but otherwise normal, and malnourished hospital patients, are equally weak. In other words 2 weeks of starvation results in very significant muscle weakness. Furthermore these two groups have great muscle fatiguability and this muscle weakness and fatiguability have implications not only for the mobilisation of patients after illness and surgery, but also for the way patients breathe. It has been known for some time that patients who are malnourished have seriously impaired respiratory function and may also have impaired cardiac function. Experiments on normal subjects undertaken some years ago revealed a 40% reduction in the hypoxic-ventilatory drive after 10 days of complete starvation.[7] Muscle weakness and reduced hypoxic-ventilatory drive are more reasons why we need to feed our critically ill patients. To assess the effect of chronic debilitation on respiratory muscle function, Arora and Rochester[8] studied 16 poorly nourished patients without pulmonary disease, and 16 well-nourished subjects matched for age and sex. Body weight, respiratory muscle strength, vital capacity, and maximal voluntary ventilation were lower in poorly nourished subjects compared to well-nourished subjects. Because malnutrition reduces both respiratory muscle strength and maximal voluntary ventilation, it may impair respiratory muscle capacity to handle increased ventilatory loads in thoracopulmonary disease.

A study by Elia et al. in 1988[9] investigated fasted normal individuals and showed that gut permeability increased in those patients who were fasted for 5–7 days. This increase in permeability was prevented by feeding subjects a mere 400 calories. The integrity of the gastrointestinal mucosa is a key element in preventing systemic absorption of enteric toxins and bacteria. In the critically ill, breakdown of gut barrier function may fuel sepsis. Malnourished patients have an increased risk of postoperative sepsis; however, the effects of malnutrition on intestinal barrier function in man are unknown. Although altered gut permeability and translocation of bacteria are different issues, it remains clear that increased gut permeability may well allow toxin absorption and ultimately stimulation of the inflammatory response. Furthermore, the adverse impact of starvation on the gut is not confined to permeability. Recoverable impairment of pancreatic exocrine function has been described; amylase, lipase, and trypsin secretion are affected.[10]

Welsh et al. investigated intestinal barrier function, endotoxin exposure, and the acute-phase cytokine response in malnourished hospitalised patients.[11] Gastrointestinal permeability was measured using the lactulose:mannitol test. Intestinal barrier function was significantly compromised although the clinical significance is unclear.

Many studies have shown that protein calorie malnutrition and micronutrient deficiencies are impaired in malnourished patients.[12] The impairment is related to the degree of malnutrition, not to the age of the patient, nor to the nature of the illness. Systematic studies have confirmed that nutrient deficiencies impair immune response and lead to frequent severe infections resulting in increased mortality, especially in children. Protein-energy malnutrition results in reduced number and functions of T-cells, phagocytic cells, and secretory immunoglobulin A antibody response. In addition, levels of many complement components are reduced. Similar findings have been reported for moderate deficiencies of individual nutrients such as trace minerals and vitamins, particularly zinc, selenium, iron, vitamins A, B6, C, and E. Nutrient supplementation stimulates immune response and may result in fewer infections, particularly in the elderly, low-birth-weight infants, and malnourished critically ill patients in hospitals.

The effect of early postoperative enteral feeding supplemented with arginine, RNA, and omega-3 fatty acids on the immune function in 85 patients undergoing surgery for upper gastrointestinal malignancies was also reported.[13] The results suggested that postoperative enteral nutrition with supplemental arginine, RNA, and omega-3 fatty acids instead of a standard enteral diet significantly improved immunological, metabolic and clinical outcomes in patients with upper gastrointestinal malignancies who were undergoing major elective surgery.

The problem of micronutrient deficiency in the context of antioxidant status may adversely affect critically ill patients. Hyperhomocysteinaemia is associated with vascular complications and vitamin deficiency. Compher et al. evaluated the relationship between vascular problems and hyperhomo-cystinaemia and vitamin deficiency.[14] Plasma total homocysteine, serum vitamin B_{12}, folate and B_6 were measured. Total homocysteine correlated with the number of thromboses. Vitamin-deficient patients had higher homocysteine levels than those without deficiency. The authors suggested that venous thrombosis is related to hyperhomocystinaemia, but it is not known whether treatment of vitamin deficiencies and associated reduction in homocysteine will reduce venous and arterial vascular complications.

Feeding and outcome

It is not surprising against this background that malnutrition adversely affects outcome from severe illness and that feeding can improve outcome. In the study by Windsor and Hill[15] it was demonstrated quite clearly that general surgical patients with protein depletion have a poor outcome in terms of respiratory complications, infection, and length of stay.

In patients on the ICU, malnutrition is related to outcome, demonstrated by Galanos et al.[16] The predictive value of body mass index (BMI = weight (kg)/height (m^2)) for mortality in seriously ill hospitalised subjects was assessed. Patients had an anticipated 6-month mortality of 50% and were stratified for BMI. A BMI in the 15th percentile or lower was associated with an excess risk of mortality within 6 months. A BMI above the 85th percentile was not significantly related to risk of mortality. This study confirms results from longitudinal epidemiological studies, that BMI is a predictor of mortality in an acutely ill population of adults. Even when controlling for multiple disease states and excluding all patients with significant prior weight loss, BMI below the 15th percentile remained a significant and independent predictor of mortality (Figure 1.1).

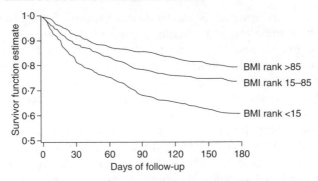

Figure 1.1 The relationship between body mass index (BMI, expressed as percentile) and subsequent mortality in severely ill hospitalised patients. Reproduced with permission from Galanos AN et al. Crit Care Med 1997; 25: 1962–8.[16]

Clinical trials investigating the potential benefits of perioperative TPN on outcome in malnourished cancer patients have yielded controversial results. In a recent study by Bozzetti et al.,[17] 90 elective surgical patients with gastric or colorectal tumors and weight loss of 10% or more of usual body weight were randomly assigned to 10 days of preoperative and 9 days of postoperative nutrition or a simple control group. Control patients did not receive preoperative nutrition but received 940 kcal non-protein plus 85 g amino acids postoperatively. Fewer complications and fewer deaths occurred in the patients receiving TPN. This study showed that preoperative TPN that is continued postoperatively is able to reduce the complications and prevent mortality in severely malnourished patients with gastrointestinal cancer.

Conclusion

In summary, if we follow patients with an illness through the ICU, nutritionally normal subjects are sick but then recover over time. However, if patients are admitted to the ICU in a malnourished state, they become sicker and take very much longer to recover. If patients are very malnourished they may not survive. Nutritional support should therefore be considered before patients ever reach the stage at which intensive care is required. Feeding may also prevent patients moving from an early stage of malnourishment to a severe stage of malnourishment. In other words we should optimise management from a nutritional point to aim for the best possible outcome.

This chapter has concentrated on the direct effect of nutrition in terms of protein-energy malnutrition, i.e. in terms of treating and preventing starvation. Earlier in this chapter the indirect effect of nutrition, through the provision of specific substrates in what is perceived to be excess

WHY FEED THE CRITICALLY ILL PATIENT?

amounts, to modify disease response, was eluded to. For example, glutamine—in relation to gut function and immune response; omega-3 fatty acids—in terms of cytokine modulation; arginine—in terms of the stimulation of anabolic hormones. These and many other modifiers are now being explored and are discussed in detail in other chapters.

References

1 Giner M. In 1995 a correlation still exists between malnutrition and poor outcome in critically ill patients. *Nutrition* 1996;**12**:23-9.
2 Jenson MB, Hessov IB. Dietary supplementation at home improves the regain of lean body mass after surgery. *Nutrition* 1997;**13**:422–30.
3 McWhirter JP, Pennington CR. Incidence and recognition of malnutrition in hospital. *Br Med J* 1994;**308**:945–8.
4 Beattie AH, Prach AT, Baxter JP, Pennington CR. A randomised controlled trial evaluating the use of enteral nutritional supplements postoperatively in malnourished surgical patients. *Gut* 2000;**46**:813–18.
5 Shaw JH, Wildbore M, Wolfe RR. Whole body protein kinetics in severely septic patients. The response to glucose infusion and total parenteral nutrition. *Ann Surg* 1987;**205**:288–94.
6 Jeejeebhoy KN. Muscle function and nutrition. *Gut* 1986;**27**:25–39.
7 Doekel RC Jr, Zwillich CW, Scoggin CH, Kryger M, Weil JV. Clinical semi-starvation: depression of hypoxic ventilatory response. *N Engl J Med* 1976;**295**:358–61.
8 Arora NS, Rochester DF. Respiratory muscle strength and maximal voluntary ventilation in undernourished patients. *Am Rev Resp Dis* 1982;**126**:5–8.
9 Elia M, Goren A, Behrens R, Barber RW, Neale G. Effect of total starvation and very low calorie diets on intestinal permeability in man. *Clin Sci* 1987;**73**:205–10.
10 Kumar R, Banks PA, George PK, Tandon BN. Early recovery of exocrine pancreatic function in adult protein-calorie malnutrition. *Gastroenterology* 1975;**68**:1593–5.
11 Welsh FK, Farmery SM, MacLennan K, *et al.* Gut barrier function in malnourished patients. *Gut* 1998;**42**:396–401.
12 Chandra RK. Nutrition and immunology: from the clinic to cellular biology and back again. *Proc Nutr Soc* 1999;**58**:681–3.
13 Daly JM, Lieberman MD, Goldfine J, Shou J, Weintraub F, Rosato EF, Lavin P. Enteral nutrition with supplemental arginine, RNA, and omega-3 fatty acids in patients after operation: immunologic, metabolic, and clinical outcome. *Surgery* 1992;**112**:56–67.
14 Compher CW, Kinosian BP, Evans-Stoner N, Huzinec J, Buzby GP. Hyperhomocysteinemia is associated with venous thrombosis in patients with short bowel syndrome. *J Parental Enter Nutr* 2001;**25**:1–7.
15 Windsor JA, Hill GL. Risk factors for post operative pneumonia: the importance of protein depletion. *Ann Surg* 1988;**17**:181–5.
16 Galanos AN, Pieper CF, Kussin PS, *et al.* Relationship of body mass index to subsequent mortality among seriously ill hospitalized patients. *Crit Care Med* 1997;**25**:1962–8.
17 Bozzetti F, Gavazzi C, Miceli R, *et al.* Perioperative total parenteral nutrition in malnourished, gastrointestinal cancer patients: a randomized, clinical trial. *J ·· Parenteral Enter Nutr* 2000;**24**:7–14.

2: What should we be feeding?

GEORGE K GRIMBLE

Introduction

Whilst this chapter addresses the question of what we should feed critically ill patients on the intensive care unit (ICU), it may be more pertinent to ask whether we should actually feed critically ill patients at all. The arguments for feeding arise from mainly circumstantial evidence that link malnutrition with poor outcome. Indeed, in 1909 Coleman described substantial weight loss in patients with typhoid fever, despite adequate food intake, associated with increased morbidity. Coleman and DuBois subsequently performed simple nitrogen and energy balance studies and came up with the surprisingly modern conclusion that such patients required about 40 kcal/kg body weight per day to prevent excessive weight loss during the febrile period.[1] Today we are also quite comfortable with the premise that patients on the ICU benefit from nutritional support. However, exactly what we should be feeding such patients for optimum recovery remains less clear.

Is nutritional support of benefit?

Several studies of hospital patients have shown them to have poor nutritional status which often worsens during hospital admission. A study by Gall et al.[2] evaluated whether food fortification and snacks could increase the energy and protein intakes of hospital patients. A control group of 82 patients admitted to medical, elderly care and orthopaedic wards ate freely from the hospital menu. These patients were calculated to be in a 300 kcal energy deficit. An intervention group of 62 patients were offered fortified food and snacks, providing an extra 22 g protein/day and 966 kcal/day in addition to the standard menu. Fortification significantly increased energy intake in the intervention group, with most effect being seen in patients with the lowest energy intake (male and female orthopaedic patients, female medical and female elderly patients), which represented

84% of all patients. The provision of fortified food and snacks increased energy intake to a level which prevented energy deficit and was thus a simple means of improving the nutritional intakes of hospital patients.

Food not only replenishes nutrient stores, it maintains anabolic drive and immune function and many other physiological processes. But does improving nutritional intake improve outcome? Delmi et al.[3] randomised 59 elderly patients with femoral neck fractures, most of whom had nutritional deficiencies on admission, to receive either a daily oral nutrition supplement (20 g protein, 254 kcal) for a mean of 32 days or no supplement. Despite being offered adequate quantities of food, nutritional requirements were not met during the hospital stay. Clinical outcome was significantly better in the supplemented group and the number of complications and deaths was also significantly lower in supplemented patients and remained so at 6 months after fracture. Hospital stay was shorter in patients who received supplements (24 days compared to 40 days). In this study the clinical outcome of elderly patients with femoral neck fracture was therefore markedly improved by a daily simple oral nutritional supplement.

Potter et al.[4] undertook a systematic review to determine whether routine oral or enteral nutritional supplementation could improve the weight, anthropometry, and survival of adult patients. Thirty studies, comprising 2062 randomised patients, published between February 1979 and July 1996 were included. Patients receiving nutritional supplementation showed consistent improvements in body weight and anthropometry compared with controls. The pooled odds ratio for death was better in supplemented patients. This review revealed that oral or enteral supplementation improved nutritional indices of adult patients, but there were insufficient data in trials rigorous enough to demonstrate whether mortality could be reduced. Benefits were not restricted to particular patient groups. However the authors recommended that further large pragmatic randomised controlled trials of routine nutritional supplementation are justified. These studies therefore show that simple measures can be taken to remedy the nutritional deficits and improve outcome in some hospitalised patients, but it is less simple in the critically ill.

The contrary view has been put equally strongly by Koretz,[5,6] who argues that the risk involved in artificial nutrition support should be considered and that one should be as rigorous in testing this mode of treatment (which consumes only 1% of the health care budget) as other more expensive treatments. Koretz's proposal that future studies should consider nutritional support versus no nutritional support is worth considering seriously because whilst there may be clinical improvement when feeding one diet rather than another, this may arise solely because the other diet is administered in a nutritionally suboptimal way. For example, several comparative trials have shown that critically ill patients fed enterally had significantly lower sepsis rates than parenterally fed

9

controls (e.g. see Kudsk et al.[7]). This seems clear cut until one considers feeding-related factors which might predispose to sepsis. Intestinal bacterial translocation arising during parenteral feeding has been widely considered to be a culprit, but a recent study has shown this not to be the case.[8] Hyperglycaemia and sepsis are closely linked,[9] and the difference between enteral and parenteral nutrition sepsis rates in earlier studies may reflect poorer glycaemic control during parenteral nutrition.

Is enteral feeding physiological?

Whilst enteral nutrition has proved to be an effective means of feeding patients, it may not always be optimal as suggested by the trial by Woodcock et al.[8] Indeed, I would contend that continuous nasal enteral feeding is unphysiological since it fails to evoke normal gastrointestinal responses as demonstrated by the series by Bowling and co-workers.[10,11] Diarrhoea complicating enteral feeding affects up to 25% of patients. Human in vivo segmental colonic perfusion was used to investigate colonic water and electrolyte movement in response to enteral feeding. Four groups of studies, six subjects per group, were performed in which low and high load polymeric enteral diet infusions were undertaken, either intragastrically or intraduodenally. Net absorption of sodium, chloride, and water throughout the colon occurred during fasting in all groups. However, there was a significant net secretion of sodium, chloride, and water in the ascending colon during low load and high load gastric feeding, and during high load duodenal feeding. This study therefore identified a marked colonic secretory response to enteral feeding-related to the site and load of the diet infusion,[10,11] which may play an important part in the pathogenesis of enteral feeding-related diarrhoea. Further studies on this secretory response showed that secretion during control diet infusion could be reversed by colonic infusion of short-chain fatty acids (SCFA).[11] This finding has implications for the management of diarrhoea related to enteral feeding, through the addition of soluble dietary fibre to enteral diets in order to stimulate SCFA production during colonic fermentation.[12]

Nasogastric feeding elicits this colonic secretory response (which seems to be involved in the aetiology of enteral feeding-related diarrhoea), whereas bolus feeding reduces it. This suggests there may be benefits if patients can be fed in a way that mimics normal meal feeding. In addition, continuous nasogastric feeding is unable to elicit normal hormonal responses. In a study of hormonal and metabolic effects of supplemental ornithine α-ketoglutarate (OKG), healthy volunteers receiving a continuous 12-hour infusion of standard enteral feed without OKG evoked very limited insulin and glucagon responses.[13]

Novel amino acids substrates

Many amino acids have been shown to have metabolic and physiological effects over and above the effects of protein feeding and are claimed to be "novel" substrates. Since this applies to 10 of the 20 amino acids, it is clearly nonsense to call them "novel", rather this highlights the fact that all amino acids are biologically active. Of those studied in depth, glutamine, OKG, branched chain amino acids and arginine seem most potent. Glutamine, addressed in detail in Chapter 6, is a fuel for cells with rapid turnover, it has roles in the immune system, it restores gut mucosal dysfunction in the rat, it reduces acidosis, it stimulates growth hormone excretion, it corrects the loss of glutamine and ribosomes in muscle, and is a precursor for nucleotide synthesis. Glutamine therefore has many important metabolic roles and has been tested in two very good trials in critically ill patients. Griffiths and co-workers[14] undertook a study using L-glutamine as the free amino acid in a total parenteral nutrition (TPN) regime. Low plasma and tissue levels of glutamine in the critically ill suggest that demand may exceed endogenous supply of this amino acid and a relative deficiency in such patients could compromise recovery and result in prolonged illness and an increase in late mortality. In the study by Griffiths et al.,[14] 84 critically ill adult patients, with acute physiological and chronic health evaluation (APACHE) II scores greater than 10, in whom enteral nutrition was contraindicated or unsuccessful, were randomised to receive a glutamine containing TPN formula, or an isonitrogenous, isoenergetic control feed. Survival at 6 months was significantly improved in those receiving glutamine TPN. In the patients receiving glutamine, total ICU and hospital costs per survivor were reduced by 50%. This study showed that in critically ill ICU patients unable to receive enteral nutrition, a glutamine-containing TPN feed improves survival at 6 months and reduces hospital costs.[14] Again using standard TPN or standard TPN supplemented with glutamine as a dipeptide, Morlion et al.[15] showed that the length of hospital stay was reduced by over 6 days in those patients receiving glutamine.

Arginine and ornithine are precursors of nitric oxide and polyamines, respectively, and have roles in permeability and adaptive responses of the gut. The liver possesses high arginase activity as an intrinsic part of urea synthesis and would consume most of the portal supply of dietary arginine. The gut reduces this possibility by converting dietary arginine to citrulline, which effectively bypasses the liver and is resynthesised to arginine in the kidney. OKG can be considered an arginine precursor. Some studies in postoperative patients have shown that both arginine and OKG promote growth hormone and insulin secretion with anabolic effects. Their intermediary metabolites glutamine and proline may also be of benefit in trauma metabolism. Animal studies suggest that arginine and OKG may improve gut mucosal function but the benefits of enteral supplementation in man are not clear (reviewed by Cynober[16]). It has been shown, however, that OKG is able to reduce the muscle glutamine deficit seen after surgery.

Hammarqvist *et al.* investigated the effects of OKG and branched chain amino acids in groups of eight patients undergoing elective cholecystectomy as a reproducible model of the effects of trauma on intermediary metabolism.[17] Patients received either a TPN solution containing a commercially available amino acid solution (control group), one containing an amino acid solution enriched with branched chain amino acids, or one supplemented with OKG, after operation. It was found that the normal postoperative loss of free glutamine from the muscle intra-cellular pool (as measured by percutaneous needle biopsy technique) was attenuated in the OKG-supplemented but not the branched-chain amino acid supplemented groups. Similar protective effects of OKG on postoperative muscle protein synthesis were observed.[17]

Nucleotides

Nucleotides have a fundamental role in the inflammatory response. Dietary nucleotides, like glutamine, have attracted attention as a key ingredient missing from nutritional formulae for many years. They are the building blocks of tissue RNA and DNA and of ATP and their presence in breast milk has stimulated research in babies which has indicated that supplementation of infant formula milk leads to improved growth and reduced susceptibility to infection. Animal studies have confirmed some of these data. In particular, dietary nucleotides modulate immune function, promote faster intestinal healing and have tropic effects on the intestine of parenterally fed rats which are similar to those resulting from glutamine supplementation, but at much lower intakes. Nucleotide supplementation has also been shown to improve some aspects of tissue recovery from ischaemia/reperfusion injury or radical resection. The intestine and liver have homeostatic mechanisms which degrade dietary sources of purines and pyrimidines (i.e. salvage) and replace it with *de novo* synthesis such that peripheral tissues receive only small amounts of nucleotides of dietary origin (reviewed by Grimble and Westwood[18]).

Underpinning the rate of synthesis of RNA synthesis in all tissues are two pathways. These are salvage of nucleotides released by intra-cellular degradation or derived from the diet, and nucleotides synthesised *de novo* from amino acids (e.g. glutamine) and sugars (glucose). The comparative importance of these two processes is not well defined, but ribosomal RNA (rRNA) production requires a high *de novo* input in cell types with the capacity for rapid proliferation and differentiation such as lymphocytes. The gut is unusual in requiring a ready arterial supply of nucleotides synthesised by hepatic *de novo* pathways. Stimulation of lymphocytes with the mitogen phytohaemaglutinin (PHA) increases RNA synthesis about 50-fold.[19] The *de novo* synthesis pathway, which is energetically expensive, increases dramatically and then switches down by about G2 phase of cell division, when the cells then acquire nucleotides from the circulation. The net result of this is that the complement of ribosomes in the cells doubles. The whole process is controlled tightly by the retinoblastoma protein, through actions on RNA polymerase activity. Measuring RNA turnover is important because of the significance of rRNA, tRNA and mRNA in tissue protein synthesis. Changes in turnover of each of these precede important cellular events such as hormone or cytokine action or cell division itself. Urinary excretion of modified nucleotides in cellular RNA can be used to calculate whole-body turnover rates of each of the major RNA species.

In a study reported by Malik et al.[20] adult patients who received enteral diets enriched in glutamine had an increased rate of degradation of ribosomal RNA (Figure 2.1). But is that beneficial? In children it has been shown that the rRNA degradation rate is suppressed during critical illness whereas the mRNA degradation rate is doubled. The rate of protein degradation in neonates with necrotising enterocolitis indicates this is also related to the rate of rRNA and tRNA.[21]

In summary, RNA turnover is a good proxy for protein turnover such that, using simple measurements in urine samples, it is possible to obtain measures of protein metabolism and the response to nutrition in the ICU. Animal studies show that an exogenous supply of nucleotides can improve liver regrowth, immune responsiveness to a microbial challenge, and gut morphology in diarrhoea models. Humans adapt to dietary nucleotide

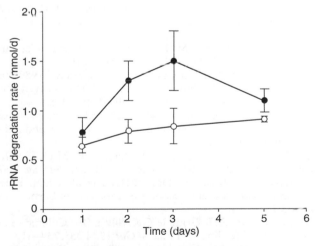

Figure 2.1 Whole-body rRNA turnover rates (mean and standard deviation) in critically ill patients receiving feed supplemented with glutamine (closed circles) or control feed (open circles). Thirteen patients were randomised to receive standard enteral formula (Protina MP, n = 7) or one supplemented with glutamine (Protina G, n = 6), providing 10.5 and 24.5 g glutamine daily, respectively. Turnover was calculated from urinary excretion of dimethylguanosine and pseudoridine (modified nucleotides in rRNA). Data are adapted from Malik et al.[20]

intake by downregulating *de novo* pathways. All TPN and most enteral formulae lack nucleotides, which may result in an inadequate supply of preformed nucleotides to gut and immune cells in the critically ill patient. Unfortunately, there are no clinical studies that answer this point at present.

Conclusion

There is much confusing evidence and although some nutritional approaches seem tempting there are few convincing clinical trials and we are forced to the conclusion that we should be performing better clinical trials to get rid of the placebo affect. Study design is clearly paramount. There are interesting new data on immunonutrition and a recent meta-analysis suggests they may indeed improve outcome.[22] Finally, a simple plea should be made for physiological considerations such as mimicking normal meal patterns in critically ill patients.

References

1   Coleman W, DuBois EF. Calorimetric observations on the metabolism of typhoid patients with and without food. *Arch Intern Med* 1915;**13**:887–938.
2   Gall MJ, Grimble GK, Reeve NJ, Thomas SJ. The effect of providing fortified meals and between meal snacks on energy and protein intake of hospital patients. *Clin Nutr* 1998;**17**:259–64.
3   Delmi M, Rapin C-H, Bengoa J-M, Delmas PD, Vasey H, Bonjour J-P. Dietary supplementation in elderly patients with fractured neck of femur. *Lancet* 1990; **335**:1013–16.
4   Potter J, Langhorne P, Roberts M. Routine protein energy supplementation in adults: systematic review. *Br Med J* 1998;**317**:495–501.
5   Koretz RL. What supports nutritional support? *Dig Dis Sci* 1984;**29**:577–88.
6   Koretz RL. Nutrition supplementation in the ICU. How critical is nutrition for the critically ill? *Am J Resp Crit Care Med* 1995;**151**:570–3.
7   Kudsk KA, Croce MA, Fabian TC, *et al.* Enteral versus parenteral feeding. Effects on septic morbidity after blunt and penetrating abdominal trauma. *Ann Surg* 1992;**215**:503–13.
8   Woodcock NP, Zeigler D, Palmer MD, Buckley P, Mitchell CJ, MacFie J. Enteral versus parenteral nutrition: a pragmatic study. *Nutrition* 2001;**17**:1–12.
9   Wolf SE, Jeschke MG, Rose JK, Desai MH, Herndon DN. Enteral feeding intolerance: an indicator of sepsis-associated mortality in burned children. *Arch Surg* 1997;**132**:1310–14.
10 Bowling TE, Raimundo AH, Grimble GK, Silk DBA. Colonic secretory effect in response to enteral feeding in humans. *Gut* 1994;**35**:1734–41.
11 Bowling TE, Raimundo AH, Grimble GK, Silk DBA. Reversal by short-chain fatty acids of colonic fluid secretion induced by enteral feeding. *Lancet* 1993; **342**:1266–8.
12 Homann HH, Kemen M, Fuessenich C, Senkal M, Zumtobel V. Reduction in diarrhea incidence by soluble fiber in patients receiving total or supplemental enteral nutrition. *J Parenteral Enter Nutr* 1994;**18**:486–90.

13 Grimble GK, Coudray-Lucas C, Payne-James JJ, Cynober L, Ziegler F, Silk DBA. Augmentation of plasma arginine and glutamine by ornithine α-ketoglutarate in healthy enterally-fed volunteers. *Proc Nutr Soc* 1992;**51**:119A (abstract).
14 Griffiths RD, Jones C, Palmer TEA. Six-month outcome of critically ill patients given glutamine-supplemented parenteral nutrition. *Nutrition* 1997;**13**:295–302.
15 Morlion BJ, Stehle P, Wachtler P, *et al.* Total parenteral nutrition with glutamine dipeptide after major abdominal surgery: a randomized, double-blind, controlled study. *Ann Surg* 1998;**227**:302–8.
16 Cynober L. Can arginine and ornithine support gut functions? *Gut* 1994;**35** (Suppl 1):S42–5.
17 Hammarqvist F, Wernerman J, Ali R, Vinnars E. Effects of an amino acid solution with either branched chain amino acids or ornithine-α-ketoglutarate on the postoperative intracellular amino acid concentration of skeletal muscle. *Br J Surg* 1990;**77**:214–18.
18 Grimble GK, Westwood OM. Nucleotides as immunomodulators in clinical nutrition. *Curr Opin Clin Nutr Metab Care* 2001;**4**:57–64.
19 Cooper HL. Studies on RNA metabolism during lymphocyte activation. *Transplant Rev* 1972;**11**:3–38.
20 Malik SB, O'Leary M, Grimble GK, Coakley D. The effect of glutamine supplementation on RNA turnover in critically-ill patients. *Proc Nutr Soc* 1999;**59**:138A (abstract).
21 Maioral LFR, Grimble GK, Malik SB, Powis MR, Opacka-Juffry J, Pierro A. The relationship between whole-body RNA and protein turnover in critically-ill children. *Proc Nutr Soc* 2001;**60**:104A (abstract).
22 Beale RJ, Bryg DJ, Bihari DJ. Immunonutrition in the critically ill: a systematic review of clinical outcome. *Crit Care Med* 1999;**27**:2799–805.

3: What route?

PAUL A O'TOOLE

Introduction

This chapter will discuss the routes that are available for feeding critically ill patients in the intensive care unit (ICU). Whether enteral feeding is preferable to parenteral nutrition in the ICU patient is, on the face of it, a very simple question and one which you would imagine could be addressed in an evidence based way. In fact when you look at the literature there are few studies, and these are difficult to combine in a meta-analysis because of a number of compounding variables. There are differences in the way feeds are used (Box 3.1); differences in the timing of feeding; differences in terms of the patient populations; and variation in the patients's pre-existing nutritional state.

Box 3.1 Problems with comparing studies

- TPN versus nothing
- TPN versus enteral feeding
- TPN as supplementation
- Timing
- Population
- Pre-morbid nutritional state

Relative advantages of enteral versus parenteral nutrition

We know from animal models that total parenteral nutrition (TPN) is not good for the gut. It results in mucosal atrophy, loss of integrity of the gut mucosal barrier, increased permeability, loss of cell architecture, and general loss of gut immunity. Both humoral and cell-mediated immunity have been shown to be affected. We know that gut flora is altered and this, along with permeability changes and loss of gut motility, is likely to promote translocation of bacterial endotoxins, which might in some way drive the processes that lead to the downward spiral of multi-organ failure.

The much publicised meta-analysis by Heyland et al. in 1998 seems to support the suggestion that critically ill patients do not benefit from TPN. These authors reviewed 26 randomised trials of 2211 patients comparing the use of TPN with standard care (usual oral diet plus intravenous dextrose) in surgical and critically ill patients.[1] When the results of these trials were aggregated, TPN had no effect on mortality. Patients who received TPN tended to have a lower complication rate, especially those with malnutrition, but overall this result was not statistically significant.

To investigate the importance of route of nutrient administration on septic complications after blunt and penetrating trauma, Kudsk et al.[2] randomised 98 patients with an abdominal trauma index of at least 15 to either enteral or parenteral feeding within 24 hours of injury. Septic morbidity was defined as pneumonia, intra-abdominal abscess, empyema, line sepsis, or fasciitis with wound dehiscence. Patients were fed nutritional formulae with almost identical amounts of fat, carbohydrate, and protein. The enteral group had significantly fewer pneumonias, intra-abdominal abscesses, and line sepsis episodes, and sustained significantly fewer infections per patient. The authors concluded that there is a significantly lower incidence of septic morbidity in patients fed enterally after blunt and penetrating trauma, with most of the significant changes occurring in the more severely injured patients. The authors also recommended that where possible the surgeon obtain enteral access at the time of initial laparotomy to assure an opportunity for enteral delivery of nutrients, particularly in the most severely injured patients.

Other studies have shown similar results, but it is important to remember that these studies deal specifically with abdominal trauma patients, who are fed via a surgically placed jejunostomy tube; the results may not translate to the more general ICU population. The other important point to bear in mind is that although the reduction in septic complications is clearly important, in nutritional intervention studies these days we are looking for reductions in length of stay and mortality, and I remain unconvinced that there are studies that show clear benefit from enteral nutrition in this respect.

The other question which creates much debate is whether or not bacterial translocation is an issue in humans. It is certainly very difficult to prove that it happens, although many studies have simply looked at venous blood to identify bacterial translocation from the gut, whereas the lymphatic system may be a better place to observe such effects—clearly impossible *in vivo*. The other difficulty in extrapolating from animal studies is that, in many of these animal models, successful preservation of gut integrity using enteral nutrition requires the intervention to be made very soon after the septic or traumatic insult, often a matter of hours. Although this is possible in animal studies it is clearly not feasible in critically ill patients on the ICU. This might go some way to explain why human studies of enteral nutrition in serious illness have failed to show benefits in terms of improved gut permeability; perhaps the interventions are not made early enough.

Of course in practice all of this is really largely irrelevant. If it were possible to feed all your patients enterally rather than parenterally—if tube feeding was simple and well tolerated—you would do it, regardless of any theoretical patient benefit because enteral feeding is cheaper and more simple to administer than TPN and of course line infections are not an issue. So the choice of enteral versus parenteral feeding essentially comes down to a very practical question of whether enteral nutrition is tolerated in critically ill patients in the ICU. Many critical care doctors still believe that it is not. We were taught in medical school that surgery is followed by a prolonged ileus, preventing the absorption of nutrients. We now know that the so-called ileus really only affects the stomach and to some extent the colon, and that small bowel activity and absorption return very quickly. We were told that we could not feed our patients until they started having bowel sounds or passed flatus and that is clearly not the case. A small study from Denmark shows what is possible.[3] Eight elderly high-risk patients underwent laparoscopically assisted colectomy under epidural analgesia, followed by early and aggressive rehabilitation. This included allowing a normal oral diet immediately after surgery. Hospital stay was reduced to 2 days without any nausea, vomiting, or ileus.

There is also a misconception that if patients have some sort of anatomical problem with the upper gastro-intestinal (GI) tract, enteral feeding is precluded due to lack of access for a nasogastric tube. This is not the case, as illustrated in Figure 3.1 by an elderly lady with a large hiatus hernia containing the whole of her stomach and some of the duodenum. She had been on TPN for 2 weeks and had suffered several line infections before I was asked to see her. It was assumed that access for enteral feeding was not possible, but I was able to negotiate the hiatus hernia endoscopically and achieve a very good tube position. The moral of this tale is that you should not underestimate the ingenuity of the endoscopist!

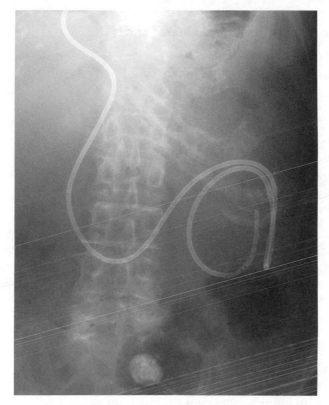

Figure 3.1 Large hiatus hernia occupying the whole of the stomach.

Potential problems

Gastroparesis

Gastroparesis (reduced motility of the stomach) is a normal part of the stress response and there is some evidence that it might be partly mediated by the peripheral effects of corticotrophin releasing hormone. It is particularly common in patients with head injury and those with burns. Other contributing factors include opioids, dopamine, hyperglycaemia, sepsis, and abdominal surgery (Box 3.2). Gastroparesis results in high residual volumes of feed in the stomach, necessitating frequent interruptions to feeding and difficulty in delivering appropriate amounts of nutrition in some patients. Aspiration of feed is a constant risk. Despite this, Zaloga and Roberts[4] have reported that in an audit of 300 patients in a medical ICU, 98% of patients could be fed within 24 hours by nasogastric feeding; the requirement for small bowel tubes or TPN was less than 2%. They achieve this is by raising the bed head, avoiding opiates, using

19

Box 3.2 Pre-disposition to gastroparesis

- Part of the stress response
- Head injury/burns
- Opioids
- Dopamine
- Hyperglycaemia
- Sepsis
- Abdominal surgery

---

prokinetic agents such as metaclopromide or erythromycin, closely monitoring residual volumes, but probably most importantly using a clearly defined systematic protocol.

Post-pyloric feeding

Sometimes, however, gastroparesis necessitates consideration of post-pyloric feeding. This approach obviously bypasses the stomach, allowing far more reliable nutrient delivery. Montecalvo *et al.*[5] studied 38 ICU patients to compare the nutritional status and rates of nosocomial pneumonia in nasogastric versus nasojejunal tube feeding. Patients were randomised to each feeding route and the two groups were similar in terms of the number of days fed, duration of ICU stay, duration of mechanical ventilation, days of antibiotic therapy, and days with fever. The jejunal group received a significantly higher percentage of their daily target calorie intake, and had greater increases in serum pre-albumin concentrations than the patients with gastric tube feeding. Nosocomial pneumonia was diagnosed clinically in two patients in the gastric tube group and in no patients in the jejunal tube group. The study concluded that patients fed by jejunal tube received better nutrient delivery, and a lower rate of pneumonia than patients fed by continuous gastric tube feeding.

The most compelling reason to use post-pyloric feeding is to try and prevent aspiration pneumonia. However, it is often said that there is little evidence to support the value of naso-enteral tubes in this respect. In my experience, post-pyloric feeding does indeed reduce aspiration pneumonia—but only if the tube is placed down far enough. In 1970 Gustke *et al.*[6] reported a study of reflux back into the stomach during perfusion of the proximal small bowel and showed that reflux was reduced when perfusate was placed directly into the jejunum, rather than the duodenum.

The ligament of Trietz appears to act as a watershed and the aim of post-pyloric tube placement should be to position the tube beyond it.

Post-pyloric tube placement

Zaloga and Roberts,[4] who were mentioned earlier, claim successful post-pyloric tube placement at the bedside in 92% of cases. However, more critical analysis reveals that only 70% of those were genuinely nasojejunal placements. Various different modifications to the bedside placement technique have been suggested. In expert hands, a success rate for blind bedside placement of 85% can be achieved, but with the less experienced, this rate drops quite dramatically. There are clearly limitations to bedside blind passage of nasojejunal tubes. If you can do it great, but if you have not got the knack the results are rather mixed. Fluoroscopically-assisted placement is much more consistently successful and is very safe. Unfortunately it commonly requires transfer of patients to the x-ray department and this may result in an hour out of the ICU, which is not ideal for such sick patients.

If the patient is having a laparotomy anyway it is very easy for the surgeon to leave a nasojejunal tube in place at the time of operation. Endoscopic placement is also straightforward; it can be performed on the ICU, takes only about 10–15 minutes and it is safe in expert hands. Unfortunately, an endoscopist is not always available when you need one and, sadly, even a relatively experienced endoscopist may not have had the necessary training to pass tubes safely. There are some contraindications to endoscopic tube placement such as recent upper GI surgery, or acute severe pancreatitis, but it is a technique that allows you to achieve very good distal tube placement (Figure 3.2).

Displacement

Even if you can get the tube to where you want it there is still the problem of displacement. As many as 40% of tubes in ICU patients become accidentally displaced. On the general ward this figure increases to 60%. Carrion et al.[7] reported a study that characterised the rates of accidental removal of endotracheal tubes, nasogastric tubes, central venous catheters, and arterial catheters. In the first phase of the study 368 nasogastric tubes were placed and 41% (73·9 per 1000 days) were removed accidentally. This was followed by a period of education and training in methods to prevent tube displacement. In the subsequent two study periods the rate of accidental tube removal was reduced to 32·4% and 25·8% respectively. The authors concluded that education of medical and nursing personnel could result in a significant reduction in patient-related removal of tubes as well as other lines and catheters.

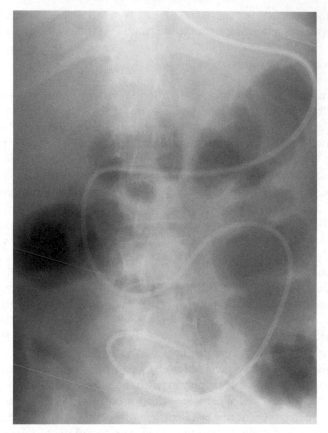

Figure 3.2 Endoscopic tube placement.

Percutaneous routes

If patients are going to need enteral nutrition for any length of time—say 4 weeks or more—the percutaneous route may be more appropriate. There are several different options.

Gastrostomy can be performed surgically, radiologically, or endoscopically. Endoscopic placement once again has the advantage that it can be achieved at the bedside in the ICU. Percutaneous endoscopic gastrostomy (PEG) placement is a relatively safe procedure, with few complications, but of course if the stomach is not working you are still going to run into problems with gastro-oesophageal reflux and aspiration.

For post-pyloric percutaneous feeding one option is surgical jejunostomy. The complication rate is around 4% but many of these complications are technical problems often attributed to surgical inexperience. Volvulus, bowel perforation, and small bowel necrosis have all been reported, sometimes with fatal results. Bowel necrosis seems to be related to impaired perfusion of the gut. If blood flow to the bowel is critically reduced it makes no sense to pour large quantities of calories into it. My own practice is to regard severe perfusion problems and marked bowel oedema as contraindications for jejunostomy.

The more common means of percutaneous post-pyloric feeding is to insert a PEG and then extend the tube into the jejunum—a J-tube or JET-PEG (jejunal extension tube-PEG). Tube-related problems (such as blockage or displacement) are frustratingly common with this technique but it is fairly easy to perform. Fluoroscopy is sometimes needed, but not always. More recently, placement of PEG tubes directly into the jejunum has been reported. The direct percutaneous endoscopic jejunostomy (DPEJ) technique seems to be fairly successful with a 72% success rate overall in one recent series of 36 patients.[8] During the mean follow-up of 107 days, no patients required reintervention for tube malfunction or displacement. Two patients developed a persistent enterocutaneous fistula following the removal of the tube, but no other procedure-related complications were noted. This is a much lower rate of reintervention than is commonly seen for JET-PEG, a fact reflected by a high level of patient satisfaction. I find DPEJ placement considerably more demanding than a standard PEG and I would rather do it in the endoscopy unit in a more controlled way than at the bedside in ICU. Furthermore, the decision to go for DPEJ placement has to be made on day one whereas with JET-PEG one can always begin with PEG and then convert if necessary.

Decision making

A lot of different options have been described: how are we going to make our decisions? Firstly, not all patients require nutritional support—but you can easily anticipate those that do. Do not waste the opportunity of that first laparotomy—get a feeding tube placed if you think your patient will need it.

The use of a clear protocol and an early decision about post-pyloric feeding is also a definite must. If post-pyloric feeding is needed then aim for jejunal tube placement and use whatever expertise is available. If you have good radiologists use them, endoscopy is also fine. If you can do it yourself so much the better. Do not miss the opportunity to put in a jejunostomy if the patient is returning to theatre for a revision laparotomy.

Finally, if all else fails, then clearly TPN is preferable to starvation. At exactly what point starvation starts to be an issue will depend on the patient's pre-morbid nutritional state and the degree of their illness-induced catabolism. If the patient is severely ill and malnourished from the start, it may be an issue from day one. Others may tolerate short periods of relative starvation without adverse consequences.

Despite the groundswell of opinion in favour of enteral nutrition, in the interest of balance and fairness it should be pointed out that the Cochrane review of nutritional studies in head injury suggested a trend in favour of TPN.[9] This is probably because TPN was generally instituted far earlier than enteral nutrition, and this may be one situation where early nutritional intervention is so crucial that it outweighs any adverse effects of TPN. This only goes to show that much more study is required in this area before we can truly say that our feeding practice in the ICU follows an evidence based approach.

References

1   Heyland DK, MacDonald S, Keefe L, Drover JW. Total parenteral nutrition in the critically ill patient: a meta-analysis. *JAMA* 1998;**280**:2013–19.
2   Kudsk KA, Croce MA, Fabian TC, *et al*. Enteral versus parenteral feeding. Effects on septic morbidity after blunt and penetrating abdominal trauma. *Ann Surg* 1992;**215**:503–11.
3   Bardram L, Funch-Jensen P, Jensen P, Crawford ME, Kehlet H. Recovery after laparoscopic colonic surgery with epidural analgesia, and early oral nutrition and mobilisation. *Lancet* 1995;**345**:763–4.
4   Zaloga GP, Roberts PR. Bedside placement of enteral feeding tubes in the intensive care unit. *Crit Care Med* 1998;**26**:987–8.
5   Montecalvo MA, Steger KA, Farber HW, *et al*. Nutritional outcome and pneumonia in critical care patients randomized to gastric versus jejunal tube feedings. The Critical Care Research Team. *Crit Care Med* 1992;**20**:1377–87.
6   Gustke RF, Varma RR, Soergel KH. Gastric reflux during perfusion of the proximal small bowel. *Gastroenterology* 1970;**59**:890–5.
7   Carrion MI, Ayuso D, Marcos M, *et al*. Accidental removal of endotracheal and nasogastric tubes and intravascular catheters. *Crit Care Med* 2000;**28**:63–6.
8   Rumalla A, Baron TH. Results of direct percutaneous endoscopic jejunostomy, an alternative method for providing jejunal feeding. *Mayo Clin Proc* 2000;**75**: 807–10.
9   Yanagawa T, Bunn F, Roberts I, Wentz R, Pierro A. Nutritional support for head-injured patients. In: *Cochrane Database of Systematic Reviews*. Issue 1. Oxford: Update Software, 2001.

4: Timing of feeding

SIMON P ALLISON

Introduction

In critically ill patients on the intensive care unit (ICU) and elsewhere, the evidence suggests that early feeding, especially in those patients who are malnourished, improves outcome. However, we should not confine our attention just to the time spent on the ICU, but consider also the whole natural history of the patient's condition. What we do early may affect what happens later in the patient's progress, and what we do in anticipation may also improve outcome. The effects of nutritional intervention in the ICU may therefore not be seen until much later.

Effects of early nutritional intervention

The subject of nutritional support for the critically ill is often divided into consideration of (i) content of feed, (ii) early or late intervention, and (iii) methods of administration, as though these were independent variables when in fact they are interdependent. Clearly, however, if you feed early but do it wrongly then the results are going to be worse. In addition, it is vital to remember that nutritional intervention does not counterbalance shortcomings in other aspects of management.

In an audit conducted by Tucker of 20 hospitals and 2500 sets of case notes in the United States, the effect of nutritional status on the average length of stay was examined.[1] There was a linear relationship between the number of malnutrition risk factors and the length of stay in hospital.[1] Of course there is a strong element of disease severity, since more severe disease confers a greater likelihood of malnutrition on admission. However, even allowing for the effects of disease there was at least a 20% nutritional component to the amount of time patients spent in hospital. The intervention effect was also interesting since the longer intervention was delayed the longer patients stayed in hospital, such that 2 days earlier intervention resulted in 1 day less in hospital.

It seems probable, therefore, that if patients suffer from malnutrition when they come into hospital, whether or not they go into the ICU, the earlier that intervention occurs the better. This premise has been accepted by paediatricians for a number of years. If feeding of premature neonates in ICU is delayed for a few hours metabolic complications are inevitable and early feeding is therefore an established paediatric practice. The small baby has very few body reserves but the question we are considering is whether it is better to intervene early or delay feeding in the adult.

Pre-emptive intervention

The earliest form of intervention is the provision of nutritional support before the onset of critical illness or any evidence of malnutrition—possible only in elective surgical patients. In a fascinating study by Nygren et al. the concept of preoperative or preinjury starvation was challenged.[2] Infusions of carbohydrates before surgery have been shown to reduce postoperative insulin resistance. This group investigated the effects of a carbohydrate drink, given shortly before surgery, on reducing postoperative insulin resistance. Sixteen patients undergoing total hip replacement were randomly assigned to preoperative oral carbohydrate administration or a placebo drink before surgery. Fourteen patients undergoing elective colorectal surgery were also studied before surgery and 24 hours postoperatively: seven were given carbohydrate and seven were fasted. In both studies, the intervention group received 800 ml of an isoosmolar carbohydrate-rich drink the evening before the operation (100 g carbohydrate), and another 400 ml (50 g carbohydrate) 2 hours prior to anaesthesia. The study showed that patients given a carbohydrate drink shortly before elective surgery displayed less insulin resistance after surgery compared to patients undergoing surgery after an overnight fast. However, not only was the metabolic response to injury reduced in terms of insulin resistance and negative nitrogen balance, but also the outcome was better in that the length of hospital stay was reduced. This work emphasises that what happens to patients before they are admitted to the ICU is likely to affect what happens subsequently.

Giving routine parenteral nutrition postoperatively is not beneficial, and may be harmful. Indeed, there is some evidence to suggest that starving the gastrointestinal tract and providing nutritional support via the parenteral route may be associated with an increased incidence of septic complications.[3,4] However, experimental and clinical evidence suggests that feeding the gut may diminish intestinal permeability to endotoxin and diminish bacterial translocation, thus reducing the cytokine drive to the generalised inflammatory response and preventing organ dysfunction.[5] The meta-analysis by Galanos et al.,[6] however, suggested that body mass index (BMI) is a predictor of mortality in an acutely ill population of adults. Even when controlling for multiple disease states and physiological variables, and removing from the analysis all patients with significant prior weight loss, a BMI below the 15th percentile remained a significant and independent predictor of mortality. Future studies, therefore, examining variables predictive of mortality, should include BMI, even in acutely ill populations with a low probability of survival. In malnourished as opposed to normally nourished patients preoperative parenteral nutrition has been shown to improve outcome.[3,4,7] Anticipating problems in the sort of surgical patients who end up in the ICU is likely to be beneficial, particularly if the patient is malnourished beforehand. Even just putting them in a metabolically fed state using a hypocaloric feed may be advantageous. It may not be possible, however, to determine with certainty the effect of nutritional intervention on outcome of patients who enter the ICU undernourished or even normally nourished for several weeks after they have left the ICU. Patients who emerge from the ICU oedematous, malnourished and with other problems continue to be at major risk subsequently.

Goals of nutritional intervention

The goals of early nutritional intervention are often not always clear. Trying to achieve a positive nitrogen balance or increases in serum albumin while patients are acutely ill are unrealistic goals which may only be achievable later, during convalescence. Realistically we should be aiming firstly for preservation of function, to enable the patient to survive a particular episode of illness; secondly for reduction of complications if possible; and thirdly for avoidance of the complications of nutritional treatment by giving too much or giving it in the wrong way.

As we have already heard, cellular function may be exquisitely sensitive to feeding in a way which is quite independent of body composition. Hill[8] studied the effect of feeding in malnourished patients after surgery for inflammatory bowel disease. These patients, who had previously lost at least 15% of their body weight, were treated with a 2-week course of enteral nutrition. Grip and respiratory muscle strength were measured and shown to improve by 10–20% in the first 7 days, long before any change in body composition became apparent. We have found similar changes in our own patients and have therefore adopted such simple bedside tests as hand grip strength, peak flow and profile of mood score (POMS) into our routine monitoring, as these are the most sensitive indicators of a positive clinical response in the post-ICU patient.

The fact that function anticipates any change in body composition is reflected in the relatively old study by Bastow et al.,[9] where the time to independent mobility after surgery for fractured necks of femur was influenced by nutritional state.[6] In well-nourished patients the time to mobility was 10 days; in moderately undernourished patients it was 12 days, reduced to 10 days by overnight nasogastric feeding supplements; in very undernourished patients the time to mobility was 23 days without nutritional supplementation and was reduced to 16 days with intervention.

It should be remembered that there is an interdependence between nutrition and other clinical aspects of the patient's condition. Serum albumin, often thought of as a measure of nutritional state, is a prime example. When 2 litres of normal saline was infused into normal volunteers,[10] the serum albumin concentration fell by 10 g/dl and remained low even after 6 hours, when the subject had only excreted one-third of the infused sodium and water. If that can happen in normal individuals, whose mechanism for excreting an excess sodium and water load appears to be rather inefficient, the implications for an injured subject with the sodium retention response to injury, are considerable. A randomised trial of usual perioperative salt and water load versus a smaller load of 2 litres of water and 75 mmol of sodium a day was undertaken by Lobo et al. (personal communication) in patients undergoing colorectal surgery. The restricted sodium/fluid group had a gastric emptying time that was virtually indistinguishable from normal, compared to the usual fluid group, one-third of whom were still vomiting by the fourth day. This also had an influence on hospital stay which was increased by 3 days in the usual fluid compared to the restricted group.

One can therefore imagine trying to enterally feed a patient in whom gastrointestinal function is impaired by the intravenous sodium and water given concurrently. In studies comparing parenteral and enteral nutrition it may therefore be naïve to assume that differences are due entirely to the route of administration of feed. The interdependence between nutrition and other interventions cannot be stressed enough.

Early enteral nutrition in the intensive care unit

There are a number of studies which have investigated early enteral nutrition in the ICU. Taylor et al. determined the effect of early enhanced enteral nutrition on clinical outcome of head injured patients.[11] Eighty-two patients requiring mechanical ventilation after head injury were randomised to receive standard enteral nutrition (gradually increased from 15 ml/h up to estimated energy and nitrogen requirements) or enhanced enteral nutrition (started at a feeding rate that met estimated energy and nitrogen requirements) from day 1. Neurological outcome was determined at 3 and 6 months after injury, and the incidence of complications was determined during the hospital stay up to 6 months. Neurological outcome at 6 months was similar in both groups, but there was a tendency for enhanced enterally fed patients to have a better neurological outcome at 3 months, fewer complications, and lower C reactive protein levels compared to standard enterally fed patients. Enhanced nutrition appeared therefore to accelerate neurological recovery and reduce both the incidence of major complications and post-injury inflammatory response (Figure 4.1).

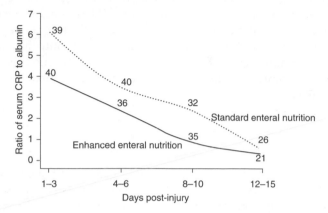

Figure 4.1 Ratio of serum concentrations of C-reactive protein (CRP) and albumin in patients randomised to receive either standard or enhanced enteral nutritional support (see text for details). Numbers indicate number of patients included at each time point. Difference in ratio was significantly different between standard and enhanced nutrition groups up to day 6 (P = 0·004). Lines are median values. Reproduced with permission from Taylor et al., Crit Care Med 1999;27:2525–31.[11]

There are also studies of nutritional intervention in liver transplant patients. Pikul investigated the effects of malnutrition in patients undergoing liver transplantation.[12] Pre-existing nutritional state was classed as normal, mild, moderate, or severe, and a clear relationship with the numbers of days on the ICU, the number of days on a ventilator, the number of days in hospital, mortality, and tracheostomy requirement was seen. Another study by Sharpe et al.[13] showed that nasojejunal tube feeding supplemented with intravenous feeding reduced hospital stay and mortality and reduced the graft rejection rate.

Beier-Holgersen and Boesby undertook a randomised double-blind prospective trial where 30 patients undergoing major abdominal surgery received a nutritional supplement and 30 patients received placebo, through a nasoduodenal feeding tube for 4 days beginning on the day of the operation.[14] Protein-calorie requirements were not met—energy intakes were only 1000–1200 kcal/day. Pre-existing nutritional status were the same in both groups. The rate of postoperative infectious complications was significantly lower in the nutrition group, showing that early enteral nutrition given to patients after major abdominal surgery may result in an imp ortant reduction in infectious complications.

Kudsk et al. also showed that early immune enhancing nutritional support in abdominal trauma patients resulted in a reduced hospital stay, less antibiotic use, and fewer intra-abdominal abscesses.[15] The authors suggested that immune enhancing diets are preferred for early enteral feeding after severe blunt and penetrating trauma in patients at risk of subsequent septic complications (see Chapters 5 and 7). Windsor *et al.* showed that, in patients with acute pancreatitis, early enteral nutrition improved disease severity scores and reduced measures of the acute-phase response compared to parenterally fed patients.[16] These data suggest that enteral rather than parenteral nutrition moderates the acute phase response, and improves disease severity and clinical outcome despite unchanged pancreatic injury. Enteral feeding therefore modulates the inflammatory and sepsis response in severe acute pancreatitis and seems clinically beneficial.[17]

Other factors

Early enteral feeding can be difficult in certain groups of patients so that nutritional requirements may not always be met (see Chapter 3). Numerous factors may impede the delivery of enteral tube feedings in the ICU. Spain *et al.* designed a prospective study to determine whether the use of an infusion protocol could improve the delivery of enteral feed.[18] It was found that critically ill patients received only 52% of their required calories. Based on these findings, a protocol that incorporated standardised procedures and limited feed interruption was designed. After extensive educational sessions, the enteral feeding protocol was implemented. Thirty-one patients in the protocol group were followed during 312 days of enteral feeding and compared with the control group of 44 patients with 339 days of feeding. Despite efforts by the nutritional support team, the infusion protocol was used in only 18 patients (58%). The main reasons for non-compliance with the protocol were physician preference and so called "system failure". When used, the infusion protocol improved delivery of calories but interruption of feeding due to residual volumes, patient intolerance, and procedures continued to be a frequent and often unavoidable problem. This study also illustrates perfectly that other aspects of management influence the success of feeding.

Another example of the interaction between feeding and other factors is seen in a recent study from a neonatal ICU. It was shown that eight out of the nine cases of necrotising enterocolitis occurred within 17 hours of infants receiving a transfusion of packed red blood cells (EA Allison, personal communication). All these premature infants were receiving enteral feeding increasing the metabolic demand on the mucosa at the same time as increased blood viscosity was reducing the blood flow through the micro-circulation, thereby predisposing to necrotising colitis.

The position in which patients are nursed (and fed) also influences outcome. Risk factors for nosocomial pneumonia, such as gastrooesophageal reflux and subsequent aspiration, can be reduced by placing the patient in the semi-recumbent body position in the ICU. Drakulovic and co workers[19] assessed whether the incidence of nosocomial pneumonia can also be reduced by this measure. Eight intubated and mechanically ventilated patients were randomly assigned to semi-recumbent ($n = 39$) or supine ($n = 47$) body position. The frequency of nosocomial pneumonia was lower in the semi-recumbent group than in the supine group. Supine body position and enteral nutrition were found to be independent risk factors for nosocomial pneumonia and the incidence was highest in patients receiving enteral nutrition in the supine body position.

Conclusion

An integrated approach to feeding critically ill patients on the ICU is paramount to a successful outcome. Timing of feeding cannot be considered in isolation. Content, route and other aspects of management are all interdependent and must be considered in a co-ordinated and rational manner.

References

1 Tucker H. Cost containment through nutrition intervention. *Clintec Nutr Rev* 1996;54:111–21.
2 Nygren J, Soop M, Thorell A, Sree Nair K, Ljungqvist O. Preoperative oral carbohydrates and postoperative insulin resistance. *Clin Nutr* 1999;18:117–20.
3 Satyanarayana R, Klein S. Clinical efficacy of perioperative nutrition support. *Curr Opin Clin Nutr Metab Care* 1998;1:51–8.
4 Veterans Affairs Total Parenteral Nutrition Study Group. Perioperative total parenteral nutrition in surgical patients. *New Engl J Med* 1991;325:525–32.
5 Guillou PJ. Enteral versus parenteral nutrition in acute pancreatitis. *Baillieres Best Pract Res Clin Gastroenterol* 1999;13:345–55.
6 Galanos AN, Pieper CF, Kussin PS, *et al*. Relationship of body mass index to subsequent mortality among seriously ill hospitalized patients. SUPPORT Investigators. The Study to Understand Prognoses and Preferences for Outcome and Risks of Treatments. *Crit Care Med* 1997;25:1962–8.
7 Von Meyenfeldt MF, Meijerink WJHJ, Rouflart MMJ, Buil-Maassen MTHJ, Soeters PB. Perioperative nutrition support: a randomised clinical trial. *Clin Nutr* 1992;11:180–6.
8 Hill GL. Disorders of Nutrition and Metabolism in General Surgery. Edinburgh: Churchill Livingstone, 1992.
9 Bastow MD, Rawlings J, Allison SP. Benefits of supplementary tube feeding after fractured neck of femur: a randomised controlled trial. *Nutrition* 1983; 11:323–6.
10 Lobo DN, Stanga Z, Simpson AD, Anderson JA, Rowlands BJ, Allison SP. The dilution and redistribution effects of rapid 2 litre infusions of 0·9% saline and 5% dextrose on haematological parameters and serum biochemistry in normal subjects: a double blind cross-over study. *Clin Science* 2001; 101:173–9.
11 Taylor SJ, Fettes SB, Jewkes C, Nelson RJ. Prospective, randomized, controlled trial to determine the effect of early enhanced enteral nutrition on clinical

outcome in mechanically ventilated patients suffering head injury. *Crit Care Med* 1999;**27**:2525–31.

12 Pikul J, Sharpe MD, Lowndes R, Ghent CN. Degree of preoperative malnutrition is predictive of postoperative morbidity and mortality in liver transplant recipients. *Transplantation* 1994;**57**:469–72.

13 Sharpe MD, Pikul J, Lowndes R, *et al.* Early enteral feeding (EEF) reduces incidence of early rejection following liver transplantation. In: *Joint Congress of Liver Transplantation, London*, 1995 (abstract).

14 Beier-Holgersen R, Boesby S. Influence of postoperative enteral nutrition on postsurgical infections. *Gut* 1996;**39**:833–5.

15 Kudsk KA, Minard G, Croce MA, *et al.* A randomized trial of isonitrogenous enteral diets after severe trauma. An immune-enhancing diet reduces septic complications. *Ann Surg* 1996;**224**:531–40.

16 Windsor AC, Kanwar S, Li AG, *et al.* Compared with parenteral nutrition, enteral feeding attenuates the acute phase response and improves disease severity in acute pancreatitis. *Gut* 1998;**42**:431–518.

17 Lobo DN, Memon MA, Allison SP, Rowlands BJ. Evolution of nutritional support in acute pancreatitis. *Br J Surg* 2000;**87**:694–707.

18 Spain DA, McClave SA, Sexton LK, *et al.* Infusion protocol improves delivery of enteral tube feeding in the critical care unit. *J Parenteral Enter Nutr* 1999;**23**:288–92.

19 Drakulovic MB, Torres A, Bauer TT, Nicolas JM, Nogue S, Ferrer M. Supine body position as a risk factor for nosocomial pneumonia in mechanically ventilated patients: a randomised trial. *Lancet* 1999;**354**:1851–8.

5: Immunonutrition

ROBERT F GRIMBLE

Introduction

The systemic inflammatory response which occurs as a result of surgery, trauma or infection may exert high metabolic demands upon patients and lead to a depletion of essential nutrient stores. Cytokines orchestrate the host response to injury and infection and are crucial for normal immune responses. Malnourished patients have a reduced capacity for cytokine production. This chapter describes the modulatory role that nutrients exert on cytokine biology, and the therapeutic strategies—termed immunonutrition—that are available to counteract these effects.

Defining immunonutrition

In my view immunonutrition can be defined as modulation of either the activity of the immune system, or modulation of the consequences of activation of the immune system, by nutrients or specific food items fed in amounts above those normally encountered in the diet. So immunonutrition is feeding immuno-active nutrients in amounts greater than the patient would normally encounter.

Immunonutrients

What are immunonutrients? Loosely, they are nutrients that have an effect on the immune system. There are many nutrients that could fall within this definition, but in this chapter I will confine the discussion to omega-3 fatty acids, sulphur-containing amino acids, arginine, and nucleotides. The omega-3 fatty acids have anti-inflammatory actions, which will help to reverse immunosuppression by downregulating eicosanoid production. Sulphur amino acids enhance antioxidant status by boosting concentrations of glutathione, one of the key antioxidants in the body. Glutamine

33

(see Chapter 6) is an important nutrient for rapidly dividing cells and helps to improve gut carrier function. Arginine stimulates nitric oxide production and growth hormone production. It therefore has an anabolic effect, and also apparently increases T helper cell numbers. Nucleotides currently have a less well defined role, but it is suspected that they have important effects upon T-cell function.

There have been a number of key meta-analyses published recently in an attempt to clarify the current status as to the efficacy of some of these compounds.[1] These studies suggest that immunonutrient mixtures, which contain one or more of omega-3 fatty acids, glutamine, arginine and nucleotides, are of benefit in specific groups of patients. However, they do not work in all patient groups, probably due to the way in which they are fed, the amounts fed, and the timing of feeding.

The host response to infection and injury

Infection and injury activate the immune system and result in pronounced metabolic changes. Immune responses are complex and co-ordinated, designed to disadvantage and destroy invading pathogens, facilitate repair of damaged tissue, and restore cell function to normal. Cytokines play a key role in initiating and controlling these responses. Cytokines are a group of low molecular weight proteins that are tightly regulated with a large degree of redundancy of action (Figure 5.1). They include the interleukins (IL), interferons (IFN), colony stimulating factors, tumour necrosis factors (TNF), chemokines, and transforming growth factors. A grouping of three cytokines, IL-1, IL-6, and TNFα, are often referred to as pro-inflammatory cytokines as they are key mediators of inflammation. Many

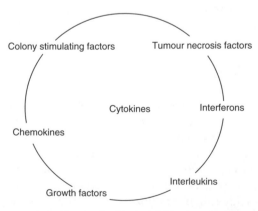

Figure 5.1 Principle groups of cytokines involved in the inflammatory response to injury and infection.

different types of cells produce IL-1, IL-6, and TNF. These include phagocytic leucocytes (polymorphonuclear leucocytes and monocytes), T and B lymphocytes, mast cells, fibroblasts, and endothelial cells. Once induced, IL-1 and TNFα are able to further stimulate their own production and also IL-6 release. Therefore, a complex network of pro-inflammatory cytokine release occurs following the initial inflammatory stimulus. In addition, indirect upregulation of pro-inflammatory cytokine production occurs: IL-1 and TNFα are potent stimulants of oxidant molecule production, in particular, nitric oxide, hydrogen peroxide, and superoxide radicals, produced by phagocytes. These oxidants enhance cytokine production. Fever, loss of appetite, and some degree of wasting are commonly seen in infected or injured patients. The wasting results in loss of tissue lipid, protein, and also micronutrients (see Chapters 1 and 8). The wasting process occurs as a result of metabolic changes that facilitate the delivery of key nutrients to the immune system, assist repair of tissues, control cytokine production, and protect healthy tissue from the effects of oxidative stress.

The mechanisms underlying these metabolic changes are complex and involve interaction between cytokines and the hypothalamus and also the direct effects of IL-1 and TNFα on peripheral tissues and liver. Increased activity of the sympathetic nervous system and stimulation of corticotrophin-releasing factor production by the effect of cytokines on the central nervous system results in increased production of glucocorticoids and catecholamines. Catecholamines, glucocorticoids, and cytokines all enhance glycogenolysis and gluconeogenesis. Both animal and clinical studies have shown that IL-1 and TNFα stimulate protein catabolism, increase glutamine synthesis, and enhance efflux of glutamine and other amino acids from tissues. *In vivo* administration of these cytokines results in rapid increases in plasma concentrations of free fatty acids and triglycerides through enhanced lipolysis in adipose tissue and increased hepatic lipogenesis. IL-1, TNFα and glucocorticoids also cause alterations in tissue zinc concentrations during inflammation and exert stimulatory effects on metallothionein synthesis. In summary, IL-1 and TNFα directly and indirectly alter metabolic processes to provide endogenous substrates for immune activity (Figure 5.2).

However, although cytokines play an important role in the response to infection and injury, they can exert damaging and even lethal effects on the host. Many studies have now shown that excessive or prolonged production of cytokines has been associated with increased morbidity and mortality in a wide range of acute and chronic inflammatory conditions. These include sepsis, acute respiratory distress syndrome, malaria, meningitis, cancer, cystic fibrosis, systemic lupus erythematosus, inflammatory bowel disease, rheumatoid arthritis, and asthma. In addition, pro-inflammatory cytokines have also been implicated in the pathogenesis of atherosclerosis, multiple sclerosis, and Alzheimer's disease.

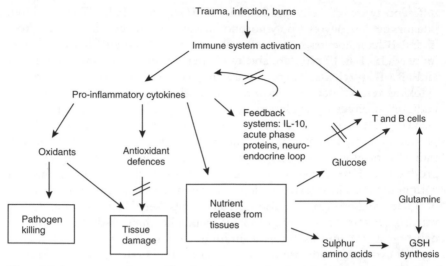

Figure 5.2 Innate systems for controlling the production and actions of pro-inflammatory cytokines.

Transcriptional regulation

Oxidant molecules upregulate cytokine production through the activation of nuclear transcription factors such as nuclear factor kappa B (NFκB), nuclear factor IL-6 (NF-IL-6), and activator protein-1 (AP-1).

Nuclear factor kappa B

The transcription factor NFκB pre-exists within cell cytoplasm in an inactive form, by virtue of its binding to an inhibitory sub-unit, termed IκB. Cellular signals induce dissociation of the IκB, to reveal a nuclear recognition site, which, after a series of phosphorylation steps, causes the NFκB sub-unit to move into the cell nucleus. Here it binds to target DNA, resulting in mRNA production and ultimately protein release. There are a large range of genes which have been shown to be regulated through NFκB; their products include cytokines, adhesion molecules, enzymes, and other inflammatory mediators. The process of dissociation and phosphorylation has a redox sensitive step, which means that oxidant molecules promote NFκB activation and antioxidants inhibit it.[2,3]

Upregulation of NFκB controls many of the cytokines implicated in the inflammatory responses seen during infection and injury. Indeed, three separate investigators have shown that increased NFκB activation in critically ill patients is associated with increased mortality rates.[4-6]

Antioxidants

In order to protect the host from oxidant damage, there is a complex array of interacting antioxidants. These antioxidants are present in body fluids and within various compartments of the cell, including cell membranes. Within plasma several antioxidant molecules derived directly from the diet are found, such as tocopherols (vitamin E), ascorbic acid (vitamin C), carotenoids (β carotene and lycopene), and catechins. In addition, proteins and peptides, such as glutathione, caeruloplasmin, albumin, and metallothionein, which are synthesised endogenously, are present. Many of these substances act as antioxidants within aqueous compartments of the cell, although vitamin E and carotene are the predominant antioxidants within cell membranes. Superoxide dismutase, catalase, glutathione peroxidase/reductase, facilitate the enzymatic processing of oxidant molecules to harmless by-products. It becomes evident that some nutrients can contribute to the body's antioxidant defences and thereby limit the ability of oxidants, released during inflammation, to activate NFκB directly or damage host tissue (Figure 5.3). Some nutrients therefore may be able to limit pathological aspects of the cytokine-mediated response to infection and injury. Many of the antioxidants act in a complementary fashion in oxidation/reduction cycling (Figure 5.4). It is also worth noting that micronutrients can influence antioxidant defences, since some of these trace elements are present in antioxidant enzymes: caeruloplasmin (copper), superoxide dismutases (copper, zinc, and manganese), and glutathione peroxidase (selenium).

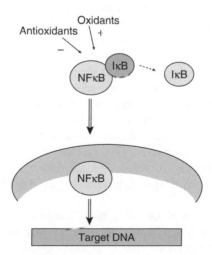

Figure 5.3 The role of oxidants and antioxidants in the activation of nuclear factor kappa B.

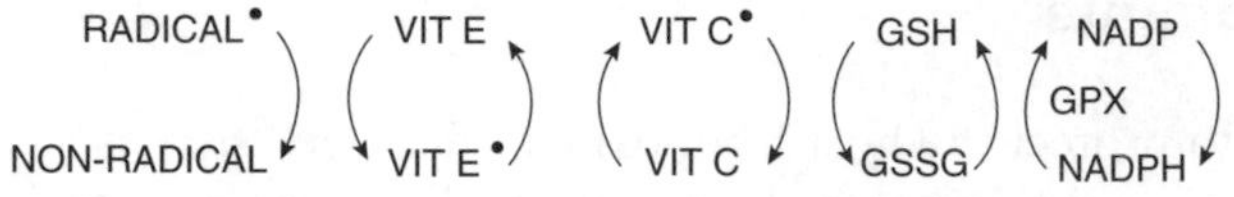

RADICAL$^\bullet$) (VIT E) (VIT C$^\bullet$) (GSH) (NADP)
NON-RADICAL   VIT E$^{\bullet/}$ VIT C   GSSG   GPX NADPH

Figure 5.4 Interactive nature of antioxidant actions. Radicals (denoted as $^\bullet$) are converted to non-radicals through recycling of vitamin E; vitamin E radicals are returned to vitamin E non-radical by conversion of ascorbic acid (vitamin C) to dehydroascorbic acid (vitamin C "radical"), which is returned to ascorbic acid via cycling of reduced and oxidised glutathione (GSH and GSSG respectively). Glutathione cycling occurs via cycling of NADP and NADPH under the action of the enzyme glutathione peroxidase (GPX).

Glutathione

Given the interaction of antioxidant defences, and the dependence within the system on oxidant cycling, it is important to consider what happens if one component of these antioxidant defences decreases in concentration. A study which investigated this, gave rats diethylmaleate, a drug that binds onto glutathione and blocks normal function.[7] Both treated and untreated animals then received similar doses of TNFα: either 25 micrograms/kg or 100 micrograms/kg. In the animals who did not receive diethylmaleate and hence had adequate antioxidant defences, mortality was zero. However, in the rats who had impaired glutathione function, mortality was 25% at the lower TNF dose and 80% at the higher dose.

Of course the question remains—does this happen in patients? We have already seen that excessive activation of NFκB confers a bad prognosis.[4-6] Another study investigated the total antioxidant potential in a group of patients with severe sepsis and secondary organ dysfunction.[8] Total antioxidant potential gives a measure of the ability of blood to quench oxidant reactions by all antioxidant sources. The study showed a large fall in total antioxidant potential with the onset of organ failure. In patients who ultimately survived, antioxidant potential returns to within the normal range, but in those who died the increase in antioxidant potential is much smaller and does not return to normal (Figure 5.5). Impairment of antioxidant defences therefore carries with it an increased risk of mortality.

Glutathione levels have been shown to be sub-optimal in a wide range of clinical conditions including human immunodeficiency virus infection, hepatitis C infection, cirrhosis, type 2 diabetes, ulcerative colitis, and myocardial infarction. It therefore seems that the normal response to trauma of any sort, and infection, results in depletion of antioxidant defences.

There are many ways of boosting glutathione synthesis (Figure 5.6). It can be achieved simply by supplying patients with the three amino acids needed to make glutathione—that is glycine, glutamic acid, and cysteine. Figure 5.6 shows how glutamine is easily converted to glutamic acid and

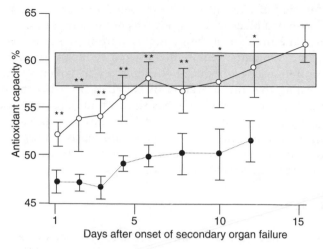

*Figure 5.5 Mean and 95% confiendence limits for plasma antioxidant capacity in survivors (n = 9) and non-survivors (n = 6) with severe sepsis. Shaded area is the 95% confidence levels for healthy volunteers. *P < 0·05 and **P < 0·01 compared to non-survivors. Reproduced with permission from* Cowley et al., Crit Care Med *1996; 24:1179–83.*[8]

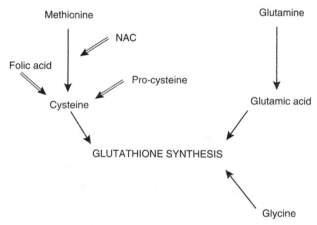

Figure 5.6 Strategies for enhancing glutathione synthesis. NAC = n-acetylcysteine; pro-cysteine (OTZ) = L-2-oxothiazolidine-4-carboxylate.

indeed this may be one of the ways in which glutamine produces its beneficial effect (see Chapter 6)—by providing glutamic acid for glutathione synthesis. It is very difficult to give cysteine and methionine to patients since they are not easily taken up by cells, but precursors of cysteine can be given. For example, cysteine can be supplied as n-acetylcysteine (NAC) or pro-cysteine.

There have been a few studies in which NAC has been used to boost intra-cellular cysteine concentration. In 1998, the effect of NAC on the early response and outcome from septic shock was reported.[9] Patients received a loading infusion of 150 mg/kg of NAC then 50 mg/kg/h for 24 hours or a similar infusion of a placebo. The study was not powered to show any effect on mortality, the number of days patients were in the intensive care unit decreased, and ventilator requirements were reduced. In another study IL-8 concentrations were reduced substantially in patients who received NAC, suggesting that the activation of NFκB is probably the underlying mechanism.[10] A more recent study has shown that the same dose of NAC as used in the previous study decreased NFκB activation and again reduced IL-8 concentrations in critically ill patients with sepsis.[11] Larger studies are clearly required to assess the effect of glutathione repletion on the high degree of mortality in patients with severe sepsis.

Fatty acids

Fatty acids may influence the ability of cells to produce cytokines and the ability of target tissues to respond to cytokines. The fatty acids in dietary fat consist of three main types according to chemical composition (Table 5.1).

Table 5.1 Fatty acids

Fatty acid type	Example	Source
Saturated fatty acids	Stearic acid, palmitic acid	Beef fat, coconut oil, butter
Mono-unsaturated fatty acids	Oleic acid	Butter, olive oil
Polyunsaturated fatty acids		
omega-3	Linolenic acid	Soya bean oil
omega-3	Eicosapentaenoic acid	Fish oils
omega-6	Linoleic acid	Corn, sunflower, safflower oils
omega-6	Gamma linolenic acid	Evening primrose oil

There have been many studies, mostly in animal models, using several of the fats. The studies have examined the effects of dietary fat on burn injury, cytokine-, and endotoxin-induced anorexia and fever, cytokine- and endotoxin-induced changes in visceral protein metabolism, and cytokine production from macrophages. In summary, fats rich in omega-3 fatty acids, or monounsaturated fatty acids, or poor in omega-6 fatty acids, reduce responsiveness to cytokines. Fats rich in omega-6 fatty acids exert the opposite effect. The exception to this rule is evening primrose oil, which, although rich in the omega-6 fatty acid linolenic acid, has an immunosuppressive effect.

The mechanism of action whereby lipids modulate the immune system is fairly straightforward. Our dietary intake of monounsaturated fatty acids or different types of polyunsaturated fatty acids dictates the fatty acid composition of membrane phospholipids in the immune cells and target tissue cells upon which cytokines act. Under the action of phospholipases, which are activated as part of the response to trauma or infection, prostaglandins and leukotrienes are produced. A wide range of physiological and metabolic changes ensue. Feeding different fatty acids will result in different profiles of released prostaglandin and leukotriene which will have some impact on the strength of the inflammatory response. A number of studies in particular have looked at fish oil (omega-3 fatty acids) as an anti-inflammatory agent. All of these studies were performed in patients with chronic inflammatory disease rather than the acute inflammation, but nevertheless hopes are high for the potential benefits in acute inflammatory conditions. Inflammatory symptoms are improved by fish oil in diseases such as rheumatoid arthritis, psoriasis, asthma, multiple sclerosis, Crohn's disease, and ulcerative colitis.[12] Fish oil reduces the ability of leucocytes from healthy subjects and rheumatoid patients to produce several pro-inflammatory cytokines and may partly explain the anti-inflammatory effects of fish oil. Fish oil also confers a degree of protection in animals against the lethal effects of endotoxin, burn injury, and bacterial infection.

Mixtures of fatty acids have also been administered, in particular "SMOF" which is a mixture of soya bean oil, olive oil, fish oil, and medium chain triglyceride oil. Schulzki *et al.* fed a group of surgical patients isonitrogenously and isocalorically with SMOF in a double-blind randomised study. Feeding SMOF reduced the ratio of leukotriene (LTB) B4 to leukotriene B5 produced by peripheral blood mononuclear cells in the patients. LTB5 is a much less potent form of leukotrienes than LTB4.[13] Hospital length of stay was reduced by 2 days in patients treated with SMOF.

Problems

A number of studies have failed to show a beneficial effect of immunonutrition. There are a number of reasons for this failure (Box 5.1).

Box 5.1 Factors affecting immunonutrition studies

- Heterogeneous patient groups
- Inappropriate end points
- Differing degrees of malnutrition
- Genotype

Probably the most obvious is the lack of homogeneity in the patient groups. Also differing degrees of malnutrition within the patient groups, inappropriate end points, and the influence of genetic variation may prevent any effect from becoming apparent.

Genetic variation

In a study by Endres *et al.* in 1989, nine healthy males were given a very high dose of (18 g) of a fish oil for 6 weeks.[14] *Ex vivo* TNFα and IL-1 production from peripheral blood mononuclear cells was decreased. However, the variability between TNFα and IL-1 release between subjects was huge. What is the reason underlying that very varied response?

In a study by Calder, mononuclear cell TNFα production was measured on four occasions in a group of volunteers (PC Calder, personal communication). Each individual had a fairly constant level of TNFα production. The subjects however fell into three groups according to the level of TNFα produced. It seems that everyone is either a high, intermediate or low producer of TNFα.

Mutations (polymorphisms) in the genes that control TNFα synthesis and release (the TNFα and TNFβ genes) have been described. These polymorphisms lead to high, medium or low production of TNFα. For example, if an individual is homozygous for the high TNFα allele (TNF2), very high levels of the cytokine are produced. Genotype has also been shown to affect patient outcome.[15] Stuber *et al.* showed that in individuals who were homozygous for a polymorphism in the TNFβ gene (TNFB2), high TNF production resulted and a mortality rate of 88% was observed. Individuals who were homozygous for the low TNFα allele (TNFB1) produced low levels of TNFα and had only 25% mortality.

Polymorphisms have been reported in the genes for other cytokines and their receptors that may have profound effects on immune responses. Preliminary data from our group suggests that not all cytokine genotypes are equally sensitive to the anti-inflammatory effects of fish oil.

Conclusion

Nutrient status has the potential to modulate cytokine biology. Nutrients may act at many cellular locations, affecting cytokine production and altering the response of target tissues to cytokines. Fatty acids can exert a direct influence by changing membrane phospholipid fatty acid composition. Nutrients which influence antioxidant defences may alter cytokine production indirectly by modulating the extent of activation of transcription factors by oxidant molecules.

In view of the genetic variability in responsiveness to immunonutrients, nutrient interventions designed to modulate the inflammatory response should thus take account of this biological phenomenon.

References

1 Standen J, Bihari D. Immunonutrition: an update. *Curr Opin Clin Nutr Met Care* 2000;**3**:149–57.

2 Schreck R, Albermann K, Baeuerle PA. Nuclear factor kappa B: an oxidative stress-responsive transcription factor of eukaryotic cells. *Free Rad Res Commun* 1992;**17**:221–37.

3 Janssen-Heininger YMW, Poynter ME, Baeuerle PA. Recent advances towards understanding redox mechanisms in the activation of nuclear factor kappa B. *Free Rad Biol Med* 2000;**28**:1317–27.

4 Bohrer H, Qiu F, Zimmermann T, *et al*. Role of NFκB in the mortality of sepsis. *J Clin Invest* 1997;**100**:972–85.

5 Paterson RL, Galley HF, Dhillon JK, Webster NR. Increased nuclear factor kappa B activation in critically ill patients who die. *Crit Care Med* 2000;**28**:1047–51.

6 Arnalich F, Garcia-Palomero E, Lopez J, *et al*. Predictive value of nuclear factor kappa B activity and plasma cytokine levels in patients with sepsis. *Infect Immun* 2000;**68**:1942–5.

7 Zimmermann RJ, Marafino BJ Jr, Chan A, Landre P, Winkelhake JL. The role of oxidant injury in tumor cell sensitivity to recombinant tumor necrosis factor in vivo. Implications for mechanisms of action. *J Immunol* 1989;**142**:1405–9.

8 Cowley HC, Bacon PJ, Goode HF, Webster NR, Jones JG, Menon DK. Plasma antioxidant potential in severe sepsis: a comparison of survivors and non-survivors. *Crit Care Med* 1996;**24**:1179–83.

9 Rank N, Michel C, Haertel C, *et al*. N-acetylcysteine increases liver blood flow and improves liver function in septic shock patients: results of a prospective, randomized, double-blind study. *Crit Care Med* 2000;**28**:3799–807.

10 Spapen H, Zhang H, Demanet C, Vleminckx W, Vincent JL, Huyghens L. Does N-acetyl-L-cysteine influence cytokine response during early human septic shock? *Chest* 1998;**113**:1616–24.

11 Paterson RL, Galley HF, Webster NR. Effect of N-actylcysteine on mononuclear leucocyte nuclear factor kappa B activation in patients with sepsis. *Br J Anaesth* 1999;**83**:170P–1P.

12 Calder PC. n-3 polyunsaturated fatty acids and cytokine production in health and disease. *Ann Nutr Metab* 1997;**41**:203–34.

13 Schulzki C, Mertes N, Wenn A, *et al*. Effects of a new type of lipid emulsion based on soybean oil, MCT, olive oil and fish oil (SMOF) in surgical patients. *Clin Nutr* 1999;**18**:27A.

14 Endres S, Ghorbani R, Kelley VE, *et al*. The effect of dietary supplementation with n-3 polyunsaturated fatty acids on the synthesis of interleukin-1 and tumor necrosis factor by mononuclear cells. *N Engl J Med* 1989;**320**:265–71.

15 Stuber F, Petersen M, Bokelmann F, Schade U. A genomic polymorphism within the tumor necrosis factor locus influences plasma tumor necrosis factor-alpha concentrations and outcome of patients with severe sepsis. *Crit Care Med* 1996;**24**:381–4.

6: Glutamine

RICHARD D GRIFFITHS

Introduction

Glutamine is synthesised and released from skeletal muscle in the systemic circulation where it acts as an inter-organ nitrogen- and carbon-transporter for intra-cellular glutamate. It is an important energy source both directly and indirectly by promotion of gluconeogenesis. It is fundamental for protein synthesis where it donates nitrogen for the synthesis of purines, pyrimidines, and nucleotides. It is necessary for antioxidant protection via glutathione, and is important for immune function including T helper cell responses and monocyte function. During critical illness, depletion of glutamate may limit these functions and may have an adverse effect on outcome. This article will address the importance of glutamine, and whether exogenous supply of glutamine in the critically ill is beneficial.

Glutamine

Glutamine is the most abundant of the free amino acids and contributes 25% to total plasma amino acids and comprises 60% of the free amino acids in muscle. It is synthesised and utilised in many tissues, with the proportion of use changing during exercise, stress, infection, or illness. Glutamine acts as an inter-organ carrier, and is the extracellular precursor for intra-cellular glutamic acid. Glutamine has a number of vital roles; it is a precursor for the synthesis of glutathione. Under the influence of glutathione reductase and glutathione peroxidase, in the presence of NADPH, oxidised and reduced glutathione are cycled, converting hydrogen peroxide to water. Glutamine is also a component of heat shock proteins, the so-called molecular chaperones which protect proteins. Glutamine is essential for cell synthesis and repair and in particular immune cell function. It also has roles in enterocyte function, synthesis of urea and glucose by the liver, and in aspects of renal metabolism.

Glutamine and the immune system

The utilisation of glutamine by cells of the immune system is higher even than that of glucose. Only 5–25% of the glutamine is oxidised; the rest is converted to glutamic acid, aspartic acid, and alanine. Functional regulation of immune cells occurs over the physiological range of levels of glutamine, i.e. plasma concentrations, such that low plasma levels will impair immune cell function. It has been shown that glutamine enhances T helper (Th1) cell responses via increased release of interleukin-2 (IL-2) and interferon gamma (IFNγ). For a comprehensive review of glutamine and Th cell activity see the review by Yaqoob and Calder.[1] Evidence also suggests that glutamine promotes respiratory mucosal immunoglobulin (Ig) A immunity through gut associated lymphoid tissue, promotes synthesis of stress proteins, and modulates apoptosis.

Depletion of glutamine

Several circumstances result in increased cellular demand for glutamine. During tissue injury and oxidative stress, additional synthesis of glutathione and heat shock proteins is required, leading to increased metabolic demand for glutamine. In addition, tissue and cell damage, for example in liver, gut, lung, or endothelial cells, will result in increased synthetic and repair function and thus increased requirements for glutamine. Activation of the immune system in response to injury or infection results in increased protein synthesis, for example cytokines and other mediators, and with it an increased demand for glutamine. During stress and trauma, the inter-organ metabolic flux of glutamine is increased due to various metabolic demands such as gluconeogenesis to maintain nitrogen and acid-base balance; additional requirements for glutamic acid are the Kreb's cycle and transamination; increased citrulline, arginine and proline needs in those tissues dependent upon glutamine as a metabolic substrate. These increased demands for glutamine are likely to result in relative glutamine deficiency. During stress and trauma, plasma glutamine levels decrease, intramuscular glutamine content decreases[2]—although glutamine synthesis may be activated, this is limited and generally inadequate. The flux of glutamine from muscle is maintained and clearance increases despite low circulating concentrations. The utilisation of glutamine within organs is increased, associated with increased glutamine clearance from plasma. Raising glutamine levels in plasma, however, does not decrease endogenous synthesis and fails to replete the muscle glutamine pool.[3]

Repletion of glutamine

Morbidity

Does the provision of supplemental exogenous glutamine have any benefit, either in terms of maintaining glutamine homeostasis or in morbidity from infection and injury? In the study by Jackson *et al.*[4] seven critically ill patients on the intensive care unit (ICU) and seven age-matched controls were given stable isotope (^{15}N)-labelled glutamine. Plasma glutamine concentrations were reduced and administration of exogenous glutamine resulted in a 92% increase in the metabolic clearance rate in the critically ill patients. Another study of 12 ICU patients, who were not malnourished, was published recently.[5] Six patients were given standard total parenteral nutrition (TPN), and the other received TPN plus 28 g exogenous glutamine. In the patients receiving glutamine, plasma glutamine levels were increased compared to standard TPN, and stable isotope studies showed increased glutamine uptake. Supplementation with glutamine has also been shown to affect morbidity. In the study by Houdjik *et al.*,[6] 60 multitrauma patients were randomised to receive glutamine enterally or a balanced placebo. The infectious morbidity was assessed on day 15. In the patients receiving glutamine, the incidence of pneumonia, bacteraemia, and sepsis was reduced (Figure 6.1). Hospital stay is also reduced with the administration of parenteral glutamine in patients undergoing abdominal surgery.[7-11]

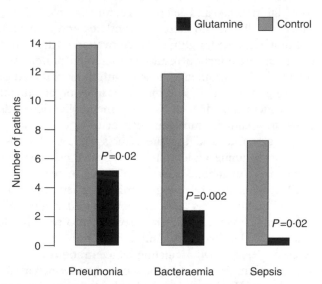

*Figure 6.1 Infectious morbidity in 31 patients receiving standard enteral nutrition (Control) and 29 patients receiving additional enteral glutamine (Glutamine). Redrawn from Houdijk et al. Lancet 1998;**352**:772–6.[6]*

Mortality

Although glutamine has been shown to both correct the deficit of glutamine, and improve morbidity, the question still remains as to whether survival is improved in the critically ill when exogenous glutamine is administered.

To answer this, it is important to know both how and when patients in the ICU die. The ability of such patients to survive infections may be the most crucial, given the role of glutamine in immune function.

Patients in the ICU die generally as a result of organ failure; early deaths from single organ failure due to the primary pathology or insult, or later deaths from secondary multiple organ failure following sepsis. The concept that repletion of glutamine might improve survival is based upon the ability to correct what is essentially a conditional deficiency. Maintaining or restoring glutamine supply will in turn maintain protective mechanisms such as antioxidant capacity and heat shock proteins and should in theory result in fewer and less invasive infections and organ recovery through promotion of cellular repair and synthesis.

The 6-month outcome of critically ill patients following glutamine-supplemented parenteral nutrition was investigated in a prospective, randomised double-blind study of 84 patients in a general ICU in Liverpool.[12] Patients had an acute physiology and chronic health evaluation (APACHE) II score of greater than 10 and were selected as being unsuitable for enteral feeding because of gastrointestinal failure due to severe sepsis. Forty-two patients received standard nutrition with some of the mixed amino acids replaced with 25 g glutamine, and 42 received a standard parenteral nutrition in isonitrogenous and isoenergetic amounts. By 10 days survival was improved in those patients receiving glutamine supplementation (Figure 6.2). The survival at 6 months was 57% in those patients receiving glutamine and 33% in those receiving standard nutrition

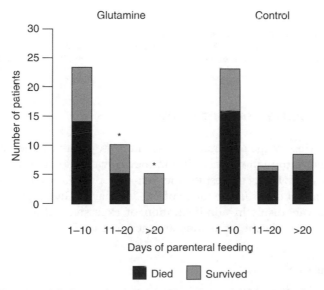

*Figure 6.2 Duration of feeding and survival in 42 patients receiving standard total parenteral nutrition (Control) and 42 patients receiving additional glutamine (Glutamine). *P < 0·03 compared to Control. Redrawn from Griffiths et al., Nutrition 1997;13:295–302.[12]*

($P = 0.049$, Figure 6.3). Subsequent studies reveal that the increase in survival seems to be due to decreased mortality from ICU-acquired infections, particularly candida.[12] There is always the question of cost: the increased survival results in a 50% reduction in costs per survivor, since there are fewer deaths with renal failure, fewer deaths with feeding, and fewer deaths from infection.[13,14]

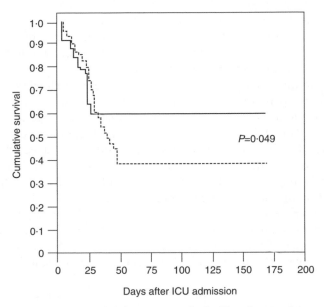

Figure 6.3 Survival plots from admission to 6 months in 42 patients receiving standard total parenteral nutrition (Control, dashed line) and 42 patients receiving additional glutamine (Glutamine, solid line). Reproduced with permission from Griffiths et al., Nutrition 1997;13:295–302.[12]

Administration of glutamine

The target dose range of glutamine used in postoperative patients is usually 12–18 g/day, although most studies in the critically ill patients on the ICU have also used 18–24 g, despite the fact that plasma levels of glutamine only increase at doses in the range of 24–36 g/day.[14] Giving glutamine as L-glutamine can result in administration of excessive volumes; the newer dipeptides with glycine or alanine are therefore preferred.

Conclusion

Requirements for glutamine are increased in critically ill patients on the ICU. There is valid scientific rationale to include glutamine in all parenteral feeds, with the lack of risk from inclusion making its continued omission unsustainable. The cost/benefit is clear.

References

1 Yaqoob P, Calder PC. Glutamine requirements of proliferating T lymphocytes. *Nutrition* 1997;**13**:646–51.
2 Vinnars E, Bergström J, Fürst P. Influence of the postoperative state on the intracellular free amino acids in human muscle tissue. *Ann Surg* 1975;**182**:665–71.
3 Palmer TEA, Griffiths RD, Jones C. Effect of parenteral L-glutamine on muscle in the very severely ill. *Nutrition* 1996;**12**:316–20.
4 Jackson NC, Carroll PV, Russell-Jones DL, Sönksen PH, Treacher DF, Umpleby AM. The metabolic consequences of critical illness: acute effects on glutamine and protein metabolism. *Am J Physiol Endocrinol Metab* 1999; **276**:E163–70.
5 Jackson NC, Carroll PV, Russell-Jones DL, Sönksen PH, Treacher DF, Umpleby AM. Effects of glutamine supplementation, GH, and IGF-1 on glutamine metabolism in critically ill patients. *Am J Physiol Endocrinol Metab* 2000;**278**:E226–33.
6 Houdijk APJ, Rijnsburger ER, Jansen J, *et al*. Randomised trial of glutamine-enriched enteral nutrition on infectious morbidity in patients with multiple trauma. *Lancet* 1998;**352**:772–6.
7 Morlion BJ, Stehle P, Wachter P, *et al*. Total parenteral nutrition with glutamine dipeptide after major abdominal surgery—a randomized, double-blind, controlled study. *Ann Surg* 1998;**227**:302–8.
8 Fürst P. Effects of supplemental parenteral L-alanyl-I-glutamine (ALA-GLN) following elective operations: a European multicentre study. *Clin Nutr* 1999;**18**:16 (abstract).
9 Jiang ZM, Cao JD, Zhu XG, *et al*. The impact of alanyl-glutamine on clinical safety, nitrogen balance, intestinal permeability, and clinical outcome in postoperative patients: a randomized, double-blind, controlled study of 120 patients. *J Parenteral Enter Nutr* 1999;**23**:S62–6.
10 Karwowska KA, Szulc R, Dworacki G, Kcromski J. Infuence of glutamine enriched parenteral nutrition on nitrogen balance and immunological status in patients undergoing elective aortic aneurysms repair. *Clin Nutr* 2000;**19**:22 (abstract).
11 Di Cosmo L, Neri A, Piccolomini A, *et al*. Glutamine supplemented TPN in major abdominal surgery. *Clin Nutr* 2000;**19**:23 (abstract).
12 Griffiths RD, Jones C, Palmer TEA. Six-month outcome of critically ill patients given glutamine supplemented parenteral nutrition. *Nutrition* 1997;**13**:295–302.
13 Griffiths RD, Allen KD, Jones C. Glutamine TPN and intensive care acquired infections. *Clin Nutr* 2000;**19**:42 (abstract).
14 Griffiths RD, Andrews F. Effects of route and dose of immunonutrition compounds. In: Kudsk K, Pichard C, eds. *Update in intensive care and emergency medicine, vol 34. From nutritional support to pharmacologic nutrition in the ICU*, Spinger-Verag, Berlin, 2000; pp. 409–24.

7: Immunonutrition with commercial formulae

DUNCAN L WYNCOLL

Introduction

Manipulation of the immune and inflammatory responses through enteral feeding has been termed immunonutrition (see Chapter 5). Three major groups of immune-enhancing ingredients have been used, including amino acids, especially arginine and glutamine; fatty acids, particularly the omega-3 fatty acids; and purine nucleotides in the form of yeast RNA. These nutrients have been combined in a number of commercial enteral feeding preparations, and the evidence for the benefit of these formulae, rather than standard feeds, to critically ill patients will form the basis of this chapter.

Immunonutrition as a general principle

The potential benefits of the individual immunonutrients are detailed elsewhere in this volume. However, theoretical benefit is not enough. What is still not entirely clear is whether there is sufficient clinical evidence to support the routine administration of immunonutrition to all critically ill patients.

There are a number of problems with many of the trials in this field. Firstly, the problem of the diversity of the patient population is an issue that appears in all studies on patients on the intensive care unit (ICU). Consequently, the mortality rates in different studies are extremely variable, ranging from 0 to 48%. Secondly, the use of appropriate outcome measures in trials of immunonutrition is also an issue. Although mortality is clearly important, the robustness of other outcome measures such as length of stay, ventilation days, and rates of infectious complications, is often contested. Thirdly, there is the problem in enteral nutrition studies of intention-to-treat analysis. Often a significant proportion of the study population may not receive the planned dose of the intervention, due to rapid recovery or death, or due to impaired gastric emptying. Finally, there has also been the suggestion that administering immunonutrients in an all embracing mixture or "soup" lacks scientific rigour. Nevertheless, probably the major problem with these commercially available mixtures is that they differ widely in composition and this makes determination of the appropriate dose and comparison of the various studies complicated.

The clinical evidence

There are now at least 30 published studies that have investigated the effects of the administration of commercial immunonutrient feeds, and the data they present are not entirely consistent. The majority of these studies have used Impact (Novartis Nutrition); two studies have used Immun-Aid (McGaw), and there are single published studies with Oxepa, Perative, Alitraq (all Ross Products Division) and Nutrison Intensive (Nutricia). At present there are no clinical data for Optimental (also Ross Products Division), Crucial (Nestle), Reconvan (Fresenius), and Stresson (also Nutricia). (See Table 7.1 for a comparison of the various commercial preparations.)

The largest enteral immunonutrition study published to date is by our group.[1] Impact was compared with an isocaloric, isonitrogenous control feed. To render the control feed isonitrogenous, it was itself supplemented with the amino acids L-serine, L-alanine, L-proline and glycine. Over a two-and-a-half year period 398 patients were enrolled in this single centre study, accounting for about 16% of all patients who were admitted to the ICU over the duration of the study. The patient population was fairly heterogeneous; the inclusion criteria were simply an acute physiological and chronic health evaluation (APACHE) II score greater than 10 points and a predicted requirement for enteral nutrition of >3 days. Although 390 patients were analysed by intent-to-treat, beneficial outcome was seen only in those patients who were defined *a priori* as successful early feeders (i.e. patients who tolerated 2·5 litres of feed in the first 72 hours after ICU admission). The enteral feeding protocol used was a relatively conservative approach with a maximum infusion rate of only 60 ml per hour for the first 24-hour period, even if the feed was well tolerated. Among those patients who actually received some feed, the group of patients who received Impact ($n = 184$) had a significantly higher APACHE II score (20·1 versus 18·5) than the patients who received control feed ($n = 185$) despite randomisation. Although such statistical analysis is not strictly appropriate, it certainly suggests that the patients who received Impact were more severely ill than control feed patients. In the sub-group of patients who were defined as early successful feeders, a statistically significant reduction in the number of hospital days and a reduction in ventilator days was seen.[1] There were no significant effects on mortality.

Table 7.1 Comparison of a selection of the immunonutrition products currently available

	Product and manufacturer								
	Alitraq (Ross)	Crucial (Nestle)	Immun-Aid (McGaw)	Impact (Novartis)	Oxepa (Ross)	Optimental (Ross)	Perative (Ross)	Reconvan (Fresenius)	Stresson (Nutricia)
Calories/ml	1·0	1·5	1·0	1·0	1·5	1·0	1·3	1·0	1·25
% Protein (g/L)	21	25	32	22	17	20	20	22	24
% Carbohydrate (g/L)	66	36	48	53	28	55	55	48	46
% Fat (g/L)	13	39	20	25	55	25	25	30	30
Arginine (g/100 kcal)	0·45	1·0	1·4	1·25	0	5·5	0·5	0·67	0·7
Glutamine (g/100 kcal)	1·4	0	0·9	0	0	0	0	1·0	1·0
Nucleotides (g/100 kcal)	0	0	0·1	0·12	0	0	0	0	0
N-3 fatty acids (g/100 kcal)	<0·1	2·4	1·1	1·7	6·3	4·8	1·2	2·9	2·4
N-6 fatty acids (g/100 kcal)	5·5	5·1	2·4	2·5	12·5	4·2	5	7·3	8·4
N-3:N-6 ratio	N/A	1:2·1	1:2·2	1:2·1	1:1·5	1:0·86	1:4·7	1:2·5	1:3·5
Carnitine and taurine	Yes	Yes	No	No	Yes	Yes	Yes	No	Yes
Osmolality (mosmol/kg)	575	490	460	375	493	560	385	320	510
Clinical studies so far	1	0	2	>20	1	1	1	0	0
						unpublished			

Another recent prospective, randomised but unblinded, study has recently been published by a Spanish group.[2] The patient population was more homogeneous than the study discussed above and comprised medical ICU patients with severe sepsis, of whom more than two-thirds had pneumonia or meningitis. Impact was compared with an established ICU feed known as Precitene Hiperproteico (PH), a high protein feed also made by Novartis Nutrition. PH has 1·22 kcal/ml, 6·62 g/100 ml of protein, 4 g/100 ml of fat and a protein/carbohydrate/fat ratio of 22 : 49 : 29. This is the only study so far that has shown a significant reduction in mortality with an immune-enhancing feed. Mortality in the IMPACT group was 17/89 compared with 28/87 in the PH group ($P<0.05$). Reduced incidence of bacteraemia and nosocomial infection was also reported.

Meta-analysis

Several meta-analyses on the effects of immunonutrition have also been published.[3-5] In the meta-analysis by Beale et al.,[3] published in *Critical Care Medicine* in 1999, trials of enteral feeds enriched with arginine with and without glutamine, purine nucleotides, and omega-3 fatty acids were included. There was wide disparity in the types of patients studied. Most of the studies used Impact but two studies used Immun-Aid. The mortality between the studies varied tremendously, from 48% mortality in the UK centre, which is actually fairly typical for severely ill patients in the ICU, to Italian elective surgical patients where there was no mortality. The meta-analysis showed no effect of immunonutrition on mortality, regardless of sub-grouping according to whether medical, surgical or trauma patients were studied. However, the meta-analysis did reveal a significant reduction in relative risk of developing an infection and reduced length of stay.

The study undertaken at Guy's Hospital[1] showed a trend towards an increased incidence of mortality in patients who received Impact. It was suggested that the reduction in incidence of infection and length of stay might be contributed to by the non-significant but increased mortality rates within this study. However, re-analysis of the data, when the patients who died were excluded, did not have any effect upon length of stay and infection rates.

The meta-analysis from Heys et al.,[4] which included only six studies of immunonutrition in patients with critical illness and cancer, found similar conclusions; no effect on mortality but a significant reduction in hospital length of stay and infectious morbidity.

Yet another meta-analysis[5] has been published in abstract form and was presented at the European Society for Intensive Care meeting in Rome in 2000. This analysis included immunonutrition studies irrespective of formulation, with some notable exceptions but also some unpublished work. Critically ill patients and both pre- and postoperative feeding studies

CRITICAL CARE FOCUS: NUTRITIONAL ISSUES

were analysed. Like the two previous meta-analyses, there was no statistical difference in mortality, but the suggestion of increased mortality in some patient subgroups. There was also the same reduction in infectious morbidity as described in the previous meta-analyses. However, the analysis appears to be heavily weighted by the unpublished study that used Optimental (Ross Products Division), an immunonutrition formulation which contains no nucleotides, the highest ratio of omega-3 and omega-6 fatty acids, and reduced quantities of arginine (Table 7.1). Further comment has to be reserved until the full paper is available.

Conclusions

These studies and meta-analyses suggest that there is likely to be benefit from enteral administration of feeds containing mixtures of immuno-nutrients in the critically ill. However, the effects are not entirely clear cut; it may be that in the future studies should be undertaken in much more homogeneous groups of patients, so that despite potentially smaller numbers of patients studied, the answers to important questions may be given.

In answer to the question, "Should immune-enhancing enteral feeds be used in the critically ill today?" the response is probably "yes". However achieving feeding success early seems to be paramount. Nevertheless, there is clearly considerable scope for more research with some of the newer formulations, regarding the issues of dosing, timing and duration of administration, and the value of particular substrates in certain patient groups. One should not assume that all preparations will necessarily have similar or even beneficial effects, so further controlled trials are imperative as new products are developed.

References

1 Atkinson S, Sieffert E, Bihari D. A prospective, randomized, double-blind, controlled clinical trial of enteral immunonutrition in the critically ill. Guy's Hospital Intensive Care Group. Crit Care Med 1998;26:1164–72.
2 Galban C, Montejo JC, Mesejo A, et al. An immune enhancing enteral diet reduces mortality rate and episodes of bacteremia in septic intensive care patients. Crit Care Med 2000;28:643–8.
3 Beale RJ, Bryg DJ, Bihari DJ. Immunonutrition in the critically ill: a systematic review of clinical outcome. Crit Care Med 1999;27:2799–805.
4 Heys SD, Walker LG, Smith I, Eremin O. Enteral nutritional supplementation with key nutrients in patients with critical illness and cancer: a meta-analysis of randomized controlled clinical trials. Ann Surg 1999;229:467–77.
5 Novak F, Heyland DK, Drover JW, Jain M. Should immunonutrition become routine in critically ill patients?: a systematic review of the evidence. Intensive Care Med 2000;26(Suppl 3):S358.

8: Micronutrients

ALAN SHENKIN

Introduction

The trace element and vitamin (micronutrient) requirements of severely ill or injured patients depend on a complex interaction of the status of the patient at the time of admission, ongoing losses, and the potential benefit of supplying large amounts of individual micronutrients. Characteristic clinical deficiency states are now relatively uncommon, but sub-clinical deficiency is of growing concern. The main effects of sub-clinical deficiency include alteration of the balance between reactive oxygen species and antioxidants, leading to oxidative damage of polyunsaturated fatty acids and nucleic acids, and possibly to increased activation of the transcription factor nuclear factor kappa B. This is associated with an increased production of cytokines and impaired immune function with an increased likelihood of infectious complications. Recent studies have indicated the clinical benefit of providing large amounts of certain micronutrients in burned and head injured patients. Further clinical studies are now required to define optimal levels of provision in different disease states, with a particular emphasis on markers of tissue function and clinical outcome.

What are micronutrients?

Micronutrients are rather arbitrarily defined as those nutrients, either vitamins or trace elements, essential in the diet in small amounts, usually in terms of milligrams per day or less. The prevention of micronutrient deficiency alone is no longer an adequate objective in micronutrient provision. New research indicates that many micronutrients are involved in a variety of aspects of cell metabolism, especially in preventing cell damage caused by free radicals produced as part of oxidative metabolism. Clinical trials of micronutrient supplements are now becoming available, so that biochemical changes can be related to physiological, immunological, and clinical endpoints. However, laboratory tests aimed at optimising the intake of micronutrients in such critically ill patients lack sensitivity and specificity.

Clinical deficiency states

Clinical manifestations of micronutrient depletion represent the endpoint of deficiency, defined as structural or functional changes that are reversible when micronutrients are repleted. Some micronutrient depletion states can present in a whole variety of different ways such that recognition of these states can sometimes be less than clear cut, although some of the changes are very consistent.[1] We know how a zinc deficiency will present clinically— the classic zinc deficiency rash can be recognised from the end of the bed,[2] typical clinical features are also characteristic of folate or vitamin B_{12} deficiency. However, for some micronutrients the presentation can be quite variable and we are not quite sure why particular patients present with a particular type of clinical deficiency syndrome.

Selenium deficiency does not present with typical classic signs and symptoms. The range of presentations encompasses simple nail changes with whitening of the nail beds, or macrocytosis.[3] The majority of patients on long-term home parenteral nutrition with minimal selenium supplementation had biochemical selenium deficiency but no obvious signs or symptoms.[4] Patients who have been found to develop clinical selenium deficiency in the intensive care unit (ICU) had a skeletal myopathy, or, very rarely, a serious cardiomyopathy,[5] like the form which is endemic in certain parts of China, where selenium deficiency occurs due to a lack of selenium in the soil. We have no idea why different patients develop different presentations.

Similar variable presentations occur with thiamine (vitamin B_1) deficiency. So-called "wet" beri-beri frequently results in high output cardiac failure; "dry" beri-beri is associated with neurological signs and the Wernicke–Korsakoff syndrome. But the course of presentation which might be of more concern in the ICU is "shoshin" beri-beri, with a much more acute onset— a severe form of thiamine deficiency presenting very rapidly with cardiac failure and severe lactic acidosis.[6] The condition is reversible within just a few hours of administration of thiamine, but is fatal if thiamine is not given.

Clinical deficiency is only one end of the spectrum. It would be extremely rare, I hope, nowadays to see patients developing these clinical deficiency states. If it does happen, usually there has been some failure to provide even basic nutritional requirements, since vitamins and trace elements are now provided in standard clinical nutritional formulations.

Sub-clinical deficiency states

Perhaps what we should be more concerned about nowadays are the sub-clinical deficiency states. Provision of micronutrients in standard feeds may be inadequate in critically ill patients with depleted reserves, such that localised deficiencies occur without overt classical clinical deficiency symptoms. The spectrum of micronutrient status ranges from optimal tissue levels through a series of steps as a result of depletion, causing changes in biochemistry, non-specific functional effects, and ultimately clinical disease and death.[7]

What we are now particularly interested in is what is happening in the middle point of this spectrum of deficiency, which can be termed sub-clinical deficiency. There are no overt signs and symptoms but biochemical abnormalities can be detected, along with non-specific physiological changes, especially in the immune system, and also in the cognitive and muscular systems.

There have been reports of hospitalised patients developing clinical thiamine deficiency, combined with much debate on the optimal supplementation of thiamine for the parenterally fed patient, particularly in the intensive therapy environment. This author was involved in a study in an ICU in Glasgow, investigating the vitamin B_1 (thiamine) status of patients with a predicted mortality of approximately 50%.[8] A retrospective study on 158 patients admitted to the ICU who required nutritional support was performed. Patients who survived had significantly higher body thiamine status than those who died ($P<0.01$). There was no difference between serum albumin concentrations of the two groups. Twenty per cent of the patients had biochemical evidence of thiamine deficiency measured as activation of erythrocyte transketolase, and the mortality rate in these patients was 72% as compared with 50% mortality overall. Follow-up results suggested that current levels of thiamine supplementation are insufficient for critically ill intravenously fed patients, although it should be emphasised that none of these patients with biochemical thiamine deficiency had signs or symptoms of clinical deficiency, that is, many of them had a sub-clinical deficiency. The authors recommended that such critically ill patients be given a loading dose of 50–250 mg thiamine on admission to the ICU.

Micronutrients and the antioxidant system

Many micronutrients have an important role in providing antioxidant protection against oxidative stress. There is considerable evidence for such oxidative stress in the critically ill—markers of free radical mediated damage are increased,[9-11] total antioxidant capacity is reduced,[12] activity of the enzyme xanthine oxidase, which catalyses the production of reactive oxygen species during ischaemia and reperfusion, is increased,[13] levels of redox reactive iron are increased,[14] individual concentrations of antioxidant vitamins are decreased, and the levels of co-factors for certain antioxidant enzymes are decreased.[9-11,15-17]

Under normal circumstances, physiological production of reactive oxygen species are controlled by a complex interacting antioxidant system, but when the balance of oxidative stress and antioxidant defences is deranged, damage can occur, targeting particularly to polyunsaturated fatty acids in cell membranes, nucleic acids, and proteins. Glutathione, vitamin E, vitamin C, and selenium (a component of glutathione peroxidase), which are probably the key antioxidants within cells, are all reduced in critical illness and also there is a reduced intake and a reduced turnover of the use of the antioxidants. If there is increased production of reactive oxygen species coupled with decreased availability of antioxidant defences, the balance is altered, and damage ensues.[18] Free radicals cause damage to cell membranes, especially to the outer cell membrane, but also to nuclear membranes and endoplasmic reticulum, and hence impairment of cell function.

Since copper, zinc and selenium are involved in antioxidant defence mechanisms, and in tissue repair and immune function, deficiencies might aggravate complications classically observed with burns. Berger et al.[19] therefore conducted a study of supplementation of these trace elements in such patients, who typically have massive cutaneous trace element losses. Ten patients with 41 ± 9% thermal burns were studied using trace element balance studies. The patients were divided into two groups of five and received either standard or greatly increased trace element intakes (4·5 mg copper, 190 micrograms selenium and 40 mg zinc daily). Energy and protein intake and wound treatment were similar in both groups. The treatment group was characterised by improved trace element status (increased serum levels and various protein indicators) and increased leucocyte counts. Of special note were the decreased markers of free radical mediated damage. Hospital stay was also reduced in patients receiving increased trace elements compared with the untreated group (45 days and 57 days respectively). Although severity of injury and wound treatment were similar in the groups, the duration of hospitalisation was lower in the treated group. These findings are clearly very promising but further studies of micronutrients and antioxidant function are required.

The study by Berger et al.[19] suggests that possibly one way of maintaining antioxidant status alone is by giving more selenium and hence reducing cellular damage. Another important study investigated the role selenium deficiency might have on certain viral infections. Beck and co-workers[20] infected selenium-deficient mice with a normally benign Coxsackie virus. Previous work from these authors' laboratory had demonstrated that selenium deficiency in the mouse results in significant heart damage from the normally benign (amyocarditic) cloned and sequenced Coxsackie virus. Furthermore, Coxsackie virus recovered from the hearts of selenium-deficient mice inoculated into selenium-adequate mice still induced significant heart damage, suggesting that the amyocarditic Coxsackie virus had mutated to a virulent phenotype.

Beck et al.[20] showed, using sequence analysis, that six nucleotide changes occurred between the virulent virus recovered from the selenium-deficient host and the benign virus. This was the first report of a specific nutritional deficiency driving changes in a viral genome, permitting an avirulent virus to acquire virulence due to genetic mutation. It is worryingly possible that a whole variety of other types of virus could also become more virulent in the presence of specific micronutrient deficiencies. Nutrient-mediated damage to host nucleotides in the short term is less likely, although patients receiving long-term nutritional support may be at risk. The role of oxidant stress and antioxidant status on nuclear factor kappa B activation and the consequences for cytokine production is discussed in detail in Chapter 5.

Micronutrients and immune function

In vitro studies have shown that most micronutrients have roles in several aspects of immune function, including T cells, B cells, natural killer cells, and macrophages.[21] Zinc is perhaps the most obvious example in this respect. Zinc deficiency affects virtually every part of the immune function (Box 8.1), including T-cell number and responses to mitogens, hypersensitivity responses, antibody responses and concentrations of thymulin, overall leading to increased susceptibility to infection in individuals who are zinc deficient. Similarly deficiencies of other trace elements such as copper, selenium, thiamine, riboflavin and folic acid, all affect immune status. Clearly, optimising the provision of micronutrients for maximal immune function becomes complicated. It is difficult enough to conduct clinical trials with macronutrients that demonstrate improved outcome in the critically ill. It is even more difficult to optimise micronutrients when the function of the micronutrients also depends upon the macronutrients. To actually observe a change in outcome, just by micronutrient trials, is difficult. However, some evidence is now available that suggests that we can optimise certain micronutrients in the critically ill to obtain a better outcome.

Box 8.1 Effects of zinc depletion on immune function

- Decreased T-cell numbers
- Decreased proliferation to mitogens
- Decreased delayed type hypersensitivity responses
- Decreased primary antibody responses
- Decreased thymulin concentrations
- Increased susceptibility to infection

Infections remain the leading cause of death after major burns. Trace elements play an important role in immunity and burn patients have been shown to suffer acute trace element depletion after injury. In a previous study[19] Berger et al. had showed that trace element supplementation was associated with increased leucocyte counts and shortened hospital stays. These workers then conducted a randomised, placebo-controlled trial that studied clinical and immune effects of trace element supplements again in burned patients.[22] Twenty patients, with $48 \pm 17\%$ burns, were studied for 30 days after injury. They were given either standard intravenous trace element intakes plus supplements (40·4 micromoles copper, 2·9 micromoles selenium, and 406 micromoles zinc) or standard trace element intakes plus placebo (20 micromoles copper, 0·4 micromoles selenium, and 100 micromoles zinc) for 8 days. Plasma copper, zinc and, selenium concentrations increased more in the supplemented group, and total leucocyte counts were higher. The number of infections per patient was significantly lower in the supplemented patients compared to placebo patients, mainly as a result of fewer pulmonary infections. A shorter hospital stay was also observed when data were normalised for burn area. Early trace element supplementation in large doses designed to meet the increased loses, therefore appears beneficial after major burns.

Another interesting study was conducted recently on patients with closed head injuries.[23] Sixty-eight patients were entered into a randomised, prospective, double-blinded controlled trial of supplemental zinc versus standard zinc therapy to study the effects of zinc supplementation on neurological recovery and nutritional/metabolic status after severe closed head injury. One month after injury, the mortality rates in the standard zinc group and the zinc-supplemented group were 26% and 12%, respectively. Glasgow Coma Scale (GCS) scores of the zinc-supplemented group were higher than those in the standard group at day 28. The groups did not differ in serum zinc concentration, weight, energy expenditure, or total urinary nitrogen excretion after hospital admission. Mean 24-hour urine zinc levels were significantly higher in the zinc-supplemented group at days 2 and 10 after injury and serum prealbumin concentrations were significantly higher in the zinc-supplemented group 3 weeks after injury. A similar pattern was found for retinol binding protein. However, despite randomisation, a significantly larger number of patients in the standard zinc group had craniotomies for evacuation of haematoma. The results of this study suggest that zinc supplementation during the immediate post-injury period is associated with an improved rate of neurological recovery and visceral protein concentrations for patients with severe closed head injury.

Another study of selenium supplementation in severe systemic inflammatory response syndrome (SIRS) was also published recently. To determine the effect of selenium replacement on morbidity and mortality in patients with SIRS, Angstwurm and co-workers[17] conducted a controlled, randomised prospective open-label pilot study of selenium replacement.

Forty-two patients on the ICU with SIRS caused by infection, and admission APACHE II scores of at least 15, were included. Patients received either selenium replacement as sodium selenite (535 micrograms for 3 days, 285 micrograms for 3 days, 155 micrograms for 3 days and then 35 micrograms per day, iv) or 35 micrograms of sodium selenite daily. Morbidity and clinical outcome was monitored by using the APACHE III score, occurrence of acute renal failure, requirement for mechanical ventilation, and hospital mortality. Blood samples on days 0, 3, 7, and 14 were analysed for serum selenium concentration and glutathione peroxidase activity.

In the patients receiving additional selenium, serum selenium levels and glutathione peroxidase activity normalised within 3 days, unlike in control patients (Figure 8.1). The APACHE III score decreased significantly in both groups but was significantly lower in the selenium group. Haemodialysis for acute renal failure was necessary in nine control patients compared with only three selenium-treated patients and serum creatinine was lower in the latter group. Overall mortality in the control group was 52% and 33·5% in the selenium group. This small study showed that short-term high-dose selenium provision in patients with SIRS seems to improve clinical outcome and to reduce the incidence of acute renal failure requiring haemodialysis.

The studies described are certainly intriguing, and begin to suggest some benefit of supplementation. All of these small studies however, quite clearly require to be repeated in different units with different investigators.

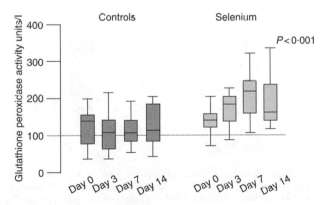

Figure 8.1 The effect of selenium supplementation on serum glutathione peroxidase activity in critically ill patients on the intensive care unit. Box and whisker plots show the median, 25th and 75th percentiles, and full range. The dotted line represents the normal range (>96 U/L). Reproduced with permission from Angstwurm et al., Crit Care Med 1999;27:1807–13.[17]

Finally, an extraordinary study from Tanaka et al.,[24] which was recently published, on the use of high-dose ascorbic acid supplementation fluid volumes, deserves a mention. The authors hypothesised that high-dose ascorbic acid (vitamin C) therapy would reduce post-burn lipid peroxidation, resuscitation fluid volume requirements, and oedema generation in severely burned patients. Thirty-seven patients with burns over more than 30% of their total body surface area, who were hospitalised within 2 hours after injury, were randomly assigned to ascorbic acid or control groups. Fluid resuscitation was performed using Ringer's lactate solution to maintain stable haemodynamic measurements and adequate urine output. In the ascorbic acid group ($n=19$), ascorbic acid (66 mg/kg per hour) was infused during the initial 24-hour study period and control patients ($n=18$) received only standard care. The 24-hour total fluid infusion volumes in the control and ascorbic acid groups were lower in the ascorbic acid group and these patients gained less weight with lower burned tissue water (Figure 8.2). Fluid retention in the second 24 hours was also significantly reduced in the ascorbic acid group. Duration of mechanical ventilation in the ascorbic acid group was less than that in the control. Serum concentrations of malondialdehyde (a marker of oxidative damage) were lower in the ascorbic acid-treated patients (Figure 8.3). In summary, administration of extremely high doses of ascorbic acid during the first 24 hours after burn injury was shown to significantly reduce resuscitation fluid volume requirements, body weight gain, and wound oedema.

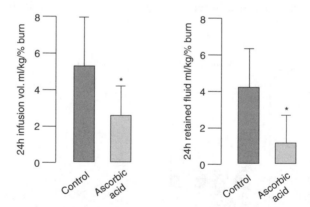

*Figure 8.2 Resuscitation fluid requirements in patients with >30% burns. Nineteen patients were randomised to receive high-dose ascorbic acid supplementation and 18 patients were controls. Data show means and standard deviations. *P < 0·05 compared to control group. Reproduced with permission from Tanaka et al., Arch Surg 2000;135:326–31 copyrighted 2000, American Medical Association.[24]*

To summarise, there have been a few studies showing beneficial effects of micronutrient supplementation in critical illness. On considering micronutrient supplements in critically ill patients several things should be taken into account. The first is the current micronutrient status in the

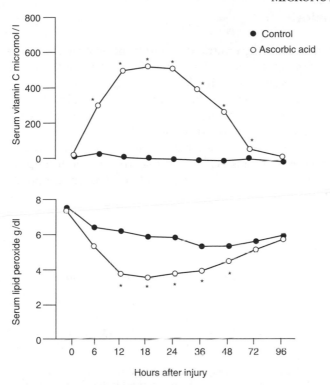

Figure 8.3 Serum ascorbic acid and lipid peroxide concentrations in patients with >30% burns in the 96 hours after injury. Nineteen patients were randomised to receive high-dose ascorbic acid supplementation and 18 patients were controls. Data show means. *P < 0·05 compared to control group. Reproduced with permission from Tanaka et al. Arch Surg 2000;135:326–31 copyrighted 2000, American Medical Association.[24]

patient, and the second is the immediate history in that patient—are they already depleted at the time they reach the ICU such that they are going to require amounts over and above standard requirements to make up for the "lost ground" over the previous period of their illness? What is the ongoing consumption? Is the patient hypermetabolic with concurrent increased requirements? Separate from the nutritional issues, there is some evidence that pharmacological doses of some of the micronutrients may be required, as has been suggested for vitamin C.[24]

Patients in the ICU are almost certainly at the upper end of the requirements for standard total parenteral nutrition (TPN) and probably require at least twice the micronutrients of a typical intravenously fed surgical patient. Some patients will have much higher requirements as a result of particular circumstances, perhaps due to burns, pancreatitis, or brain injury.[25] Many of the pharmaceutical companies are beginning to look at the special requirements of the intensive care patient, and this is certainly an area in which developments will be seen over the next year or two.

Conclusions

There are increased micronutrient requirements in critical illness, particularly as a result of increased metabolic stresses, but also because these patients will have various losses from the body, through dialysis, fistulae, etc. The assessment of requirements is almost impossible using laboratory tests due to the non-specificity of such tests, such that clinical judgement as to what the requirements are likely to be in the individual patients is the only practical suggestion. However if adequate—and probably even excessive—micronutrient provision is achieved it may be possible to improve outcome, but more clinical trials with clinical outcome as an endpoint are clearly needed.

References

1   McLaren DS. *A Colour Atlas and Text of Diet-Related Disorders*, 2nd ed London: Mosby Year Book Europe Limited, 1992.
2   Kay RG, Tasman-Jones C, Pybus J, *et al*. A syndrome of acute zinc deficiency during total parenteral alimentation in man. *Ann Surg* 1976;**183**:331–40.
3   Vinton N, Dahlstrom K, Stroblel CT, Ament M. Macrocytosis and pseudoalbinism: manifestations of selenium deficiency. *Paediatrics* 1988;**111**:711–17.
4   Shenkin A, Fell GS, Halls DJ, *et al*. Essential trace element provision to patients receiving home intravenous nutrition in the United Kingdom. *Clin Nutr* 1986; **5**:91–7.
5   Johnson RA, Baker SS, Fallon JT, *et al*. An accidental case of cardiomyopathy and selenium deficiency. *N Engl J Med* 1981;**304**:1210–12.
6   La Selve P, Demolin P, Holzapfel L, *et al*. Shoshin beriberi: an unusual complication of prolonged parenteral nutrition. *J Parenteral Enter Nutr* 1986;**10**:102–3.
7   Shenkin A. Micronutrients in the severely-injured patient. *Proc Nutr Soc* 2000; **59**:451–56.
8   Cruickshank AM, Telfer AB, Shenkin A. Thiamine deficiency in the critically ill. *Intensive Care Med* 1988;**14**:384–7.
9   Cross CE, Forte T, Stocker R, *et al*. Oxidative stress and abnormal cholesterol metabolism in patients with adult respiratory distress syndrome. *J Lab Clin Med* 1990;**115**:396–404.
10 Takeda K, Shimada Y, Amano M, Sakai T, Okada T, Yoshiya I. Plasma lipid peroxides and alpha-tocopherol in critically ill patients. *Crit Care Med* 1984; **12**:957–9.
11 Richard C, Lemonnier F, Thibault M, Couturier M, Auzepy P. Vitamin E deficiency and lipoperoxidation during adult respiratory distress syndrome. *Crit Care Med* 1990;**18**:4–9.
12 Cowley HC, Bacon PJ, Goode HF, Webster NR, Jones JG, Menon DK. Plasma antioxidant potential in severe sepsis: a comparison of survivors and nonsurvivors. *Crit Care Med* 1996;**24**:1179–83.
13 Galley HF, Davies MJ, Webster NR. Xanthine oxidase activity and free radical generation in patients with sepsis syndrome. *Crit Care Med* 1996;**24**:1649–53.

14 Galley HF, Webster NR. Elevated serum bleomycin-detectable iron concentrations in patients with sepsis syndrome. *Intensive Care Med* 1996;**22**:226–9.

15 Schorah CJ, Downing C, Piripitso A, *et al.* Total vitamin C, ascorbic acid, and dehydroascorbic acid concentrations in plasma of critically ill patients. *Am J Clin Nutr* 1996;**63**:760–5.

16 Borrelli E, Roux-Lombard P, Grau GE, *et al.* Plasma concentrations of cytokines, their soluble receptors, and antioxidant vitamins can predict the development of multiple organ failure in patients at risk. *Crit Care Med* 1996; **24**:392–7.

17 Angstwurm MW, Schottdorf J, Schopohl J, Gaertner R. Selenium replacement in patients with severe systemic inflammatory response syndrome improves clinical outcome. *Crit Care Med* 1999;**27**:1807–13.

18 Borhani M, Helton WS. Antioxidants in critical illness. In: Pichard C, Kudsk KA, eds. *From Nutrition Support to Pharmacologic Nutrition in the ICU. Update in Intensive Care and Emergency Medicine*, 34. Berlin: Springer, 2000;80–91.

19 Berger MM, Cavadini C, Chiolero R, Guinchard S, Krupp S, Dirren H. Influence of large intakes of trace elements on recovery after major burns. *Nutrition* 1994;**10**:327–34.

20 Beck MA, Shi Q, Morris VC, Levander OA. Rapid genomic evolution of a non-virulent coxsackievirus B3 in selenium-deficient mice results in selection of identical virulent isolates. *Nat Med* 1995;**1**:433–6.

21 Chandra RK. Nutrition and the immune system: an introduction. *Am J Clin Nutr* 1997;**66**:460S–3S.

22 Berger MM, Spertini F, Shenkin A, *et al.* Trace element supplementation modulates pulmonary infection rates after major burns: a double-blind, placebo-controlled trial. *Am J Clin Nutr* 1998;**68**:365–71.

23 Young B, Ott L, Kasarskis E, *et al.* Zinc supplementation is associated with improved neurologic recovery rate and visceral protein levels of patients with severe closed head injury. *J Neurotrauma* 1996;**13**:25–34.

24 Tanaka H, Matsuda T, Miyagantani Y, Yukioka T, Matsuda H, Shimazaki S. Reduction of resuscitation fluid volumes in severely burned patients using ascorbic acid administration: a randomized, prospective study. *Arch Surg* 2000; **135**:326–31.

25 Berger MM, Shenkin A. Trace elements in vitamins. In: Pichard C, Kudsk KA, eds. *From Nutrition Support to Pharmacologic Nutrition in the ICU. Update in Intensive Care and Emergency Medicine*, 34. Berlin: Springer, 2000;66–79.

Index

INDEX